D1601702

Debating Your Plate

The Most Controversial Foods and Ingredients

Randi Minetor

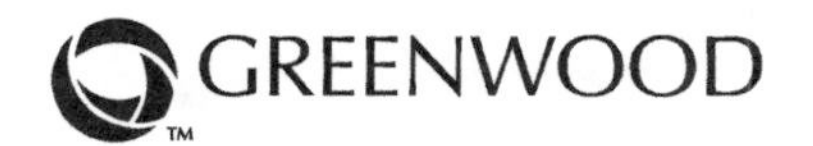

An Imprint of ABC-CLIO, LLC
Santa Barbara, California • Denver, Colorado

Library of Congress Cataloging-in-Publication Data

Names: Minetor, Randi, author.
Title: Debating your plate : the most controversial foods and ingredients / Randi Minetor.
Description: 1st edition. | Santa Barbara, California : Greenwood, [2022] | Includes bibliographical references and index.
Identifiers: LCCN 2021009692 (print) | LCCN 2021009693 (ebook) | ISBN 9781440874352 (hardcover) | ISBN 9781440874369 (ebook)
Subjects: LCSH: Nutrition. | Food preferences. | Diet. | Food habits.
Classification: LCC RA784 .M51512 2022 (print) | LCC RA784 (ebook) | DDC 613.2—dc23
LC record available at https://lccn.loc.gov/2021009692
LC ebook record available at https://lccn.loc.gov/2021009693

ISBN: 978-1-4408-7435-2 (print)
978-1-4408-7436-9 (ebook)

26 25 24 23 22 1 2 3 4 5

This book is also available as an eBook.

Greenwood
An Imprint of ABC-CLIO, LLC

ABC-CLIO, LLC
147 Castilian Drive
Santa Barbara, California 93117
www.abc-clio.com

This book is printed on acid-free paper ∞

Manufactured in the United States of America

Contents

Introduction

"An apple a day keeps the doctor away," the old proverb goes, one that every kindergartener has recited for more than a century, and few people would argue that apples are not a healthy snack. It may surprise readers to learn that this saying did not originally spring from the marketing department of an apple growers' association. In fact, the original aphorism comes from the Welsh town of Pembrokeshire and first appeared in print in 1866: "Eat an apple on going to bed, and you'll keep the doctor from earning his bread."

Chances are that most parents do not take the apple prescription as medical advice, but the saying may give them enough pause that they select a shiny red apple for their child's lunch bag instead of a pack of cookies. This may be considered a positive outcome, but it tells us a great deal about how we choose what we eat and whether we can and should trust the information presented to us as facts without knowing its origins.

Innocent enough on the face of it, the apple-a-day expression made its way into the public consciousness and solidified its place there without a scrap of evidence to support its lofty claim. Apples became so synonymous with good health practices that in 2015, a team of three researchers at Dartmouth's Geisel School of Medicine, the University of Michigan, and the Veteran Affairs Medical Center Outcomes Group completed an actual study "to examine the relationship between eating an apple a day and keeping the doctor away."

Can you guess what they found? Some 8,399 study participants filled out a dietary recall questionnaire, and just 9 percent of these turned out to be regular apple eaters. Comparing apple consumers with the others, the researchers reported no statistical significance between eating apples and the number of doctor visits, overnight hospital stays, or mental health visits the participants reported. The only real difference, the study concluded, was in the need for prescription medications: Apple eaters seemed to use fewer medications than those who did not eat apples.

"Through the ages, the apple has come to symbolize health and healthy habits, and has been used by government and private health organizations to symbolize lifestyle choices that lead to health and wellness," the researchers reported. This place in a balanced diet has not come about because the apple has some special health-giving property, but because its namesake proverb has been "promoted by the lay media and powerful special interest groups, including the U.S. Apple Association."

Most consumers will not parse their way through medical journals to find the studies that support or refute the claims of advertising slogans, but they may read websites, skim magazine articles, and watch videos and television news stories that take such research and boil it down to its essence. Some of these misinterpret the studies they cover, while others oversimplify the results. Still others convolute the information to serve their own purposes or to promote a specific diet or lifestyle as the answer to permanent weight loss and good health. And many others, especially special interest groups working for food industries, pay for research to be sure that it places their product in a positive spotlight.

Debating Your Plate provides an overview of the ways in which influencers guide messages about the thousands of food choices presented to us and how these messages may mislead us. This book traces well-vetted research, questionable studies, marketing campaigns, biased and unbiased reporting, and media hype in an attempt to find some kernel of truth still remaining among the noise.

I am a journalist, not a scientist, so I cannot draw final conclusions for readers; but I have presented as many sides to each discussion as I could find to help you become a more educated consumer of food industry information. If, in the end, you make healthier and more informed choices for your own plate, this book has done its job.

As you will see from the Contents, the foods and food additives chosen here are those for which controversy continues, not those that have become matters of settled science. We know, for example, that trans fats are particularly harmful to the human body, and lawmakers have gone so far as to ban them in some U.S. regions. There is no need to debate this further, so trans fats, while mentioned in passing, do not get their own chapter. Nor does high-fructose corn syrup, another well-understood sweetener linked to many serious health issues. You will find a discussion of sugar in a section titled "The History of Food Controversies" and again in the chapter about fruit juices, but this book delves more directly into the question of artificial sweeteners and sugar alcohols, two hotly debated classes of ingredients.

In a world where information from multiple sources bombards every consumer, we need to be vigilant about what we accept as fact and what is obviously meant to fool us. *Debating Your Plate* takes on a subject that affects every human being, helps you look beyond the headlines, and finds what you really need to know about the food you eat.

RESOURCE

Davis, Matthew A., et al. "Association Between Apple Consumption and Physician Visits." *JAMA Internal Medicine*, May 1, 2015, 175(5), 777–783. Accessed Jan. 19, 2020. https://www.ncbi.nlm.nih.gov/pmc/articles/PMC4420713

Why Is Nutrition So Controversial?

Hardly a day goes by without a new study emerging in the media, telling us that something is wrong with our food. A choice we believed to be healthy actually has the potential to ruin our good health. A favorite food turns out to be loaded with ingredients we already knew had to be consumed in moderation, tipping the scales toward harm if we dare to have an extra cookie or a second helping of potatoes.

Experts, some legitimate and some self-proclaimed, tell us to consume more "superfoods," but the list of these foods has become a moving target, with new, exotic-sounding ingredients rising to public consciousness on a regular basis. Unfamiliar fruits, vegetables, and grains are hailed as miraculous health-builders with the ability to prevent cancer, heart disease, diabetes, and more. Magazines and online articles urge people to cast away the foods we have eaten for centuries in favor of acai berries, goji berries, quinoa, freekeh, farro, bulgur, einkorn, spirulina, mangosteen, bee pollen, maca root, and many others—often long before science has caught up with these and other foodstuffs. Will this shift actually produce the promised results? Researchers rarely have the opportunity to delve into these claims before the ingredients arrive on store shelves, so marketers of these wonder foods may be the only ones to tout their superiority. Consumers looking for magical health boosts may frequent stores that specialize in nutritional supplements or take the word of a personal trainer or health-club owner, rather than seek the peer-reviewed science that might support or negate their claims.

Here in the twenty-first century, it seems that something as basic as proper nutrition should be settled science. The *2015–2020 Dietary Guidelines for Americans* (DGA), a publication based on decades of scientific research and published by the U.S. Department of Agriculture, provides sound nutritional advice that seems simple enough for households to follow. There is even a website, ChooseMyPlate.gov, that helps consumers build their own meal plan. Yet even as it provides the advice we need to pursue an informed diet and achieve lifelong health, the DGA notes that as many as half of all American adults live with chronic diseases related directly to the low quality of their dietary choices. What percentage of these people truly have no access to fresh foods and healthy choices and which are simply fast-food lovers cannot be gleaned easily from media reports and studies. We do know that 117 million people in the United States alone live with cardiovascular disease, high blood pressure, type 2 diabetes, cancer, and bone disease, all of which can be attributed directly to the foods they eat.

"More than two-thirds of adults and nearly one-third of children and youth are overweight or obese," the DGA's introduction tells us:

> These high rates of overweight and obesity and chronic disease have persisted for more than two decades and come not only with increased health risks, but also at high cost. In 2008, the medical costs associated with obesity were estimated to be $147 billion. In 2012, the total estimated cost of diagnosed diabetes was $245 billion, including $176 billion in direct medical costs and $69 billion in decreased productivity.

So eating the wrong foods is making us sick, and these sicknesses are costing the American people a fortune. Is the DGA so difficult to understand that people can't decipher it? Aren't doctors giving this information to their patients to help them improve their own health? Or is something else afoot?

Let's take a look at what the guidelines call a healthy "eating pattern"—the foods that people tend to choose to eat and drink on a daily or weekly basis. A healthy eating pattern includes "all foods and beverages within an appropriate caloric level," so an awareness of what constitutes a serving of each food becomes a critical component of balanced nutrition.

Here are the elements of a healthy eating pattern named in the DGA:

- Vegetables, with varieties including dark green, red, and orange, starchy, and legumes (beans and peas)
- Fruits, including 100 percent fruit juices with no added sugar
- Grains, with whole grains making up half of all grains consumed
- Dairy—but only the fat-free or low-fat products, and including soy beverages
- Proteins, including fish and other seafood, lean meats, lean poultry, eggs, nuts, legumes, seeds, and soy products
- Oils of the monosaturated or polyunsaturated varieties

So far, it's likely that nothing on this list comes as a surprise. We know that eating whole fruits and vegetables is a healthy choice, and wholesome grains, lean meats, poultry, and fish (or beans and nuts for vegetarians and vegans) are known elements in a well-rounded diet.

The DGA continues, however, by setting significant limits on saturated fats, trans fats—the fats created by adding hydrogen to vegetable oil—sugar, and salt (sodium). These limits have been set using well-documented, peer-reviewed science that shows us that too much of these substances have a negative impact on human health.

- Saturated fats are solid at room temperature and include the fat that marbles red meats, the fat found under the skin of poultry, and the fat in cream, lard, butter, full-fat cheese, and whole milk. The DGA recommends that we keep saturated fats down to 10 percent or less of our daily calories.
- Trans fats, also known as trans-fatty acids, are largely created by an industrial process so that they retain their solid consistency at room temperature. This makes them last longer on the shelf than monosaturated and polyunsaturated fats, two kinds of fat that are necessary (in moderation) for a healthy diet. Trans fats increase the body's LDL cholesterol—the bad kind—while lowering the good HDL cholesterol in a destructive double-punch to the human system. The Food and Drug Administration (FDA) recommends that we avoid products that use trans fats (look for "partially hydrogenated" in the ingredients list on packaged products and a trans fat listing in the nutritional breakdown). Most food packagers have stopped using them, but products including vegetable shortening, some microwave popcorn, some margarines and vegetable oils, fried fast foods, bakery products, canned frosting, piecrusts, nondairy coffee creamers, and some snacks still contain them.
- The sugar added to processed foods—soft drinks, energy drinks, candy, cookies and other baked goods, flavored yogurt, ice cream, cereals, and some soups, bread, ketchup, processed meats, and so on—gets processed in the liver, which can be overwhelmed when a person consumes too much sugar. This leads to weight gain, fatty liver disease, high blood pressure, heart disease, and diabetes—and eventually to heart attack and stroke. The guidelines recommend that we consume less than 10 percent of our daily calories from added sugar.
- The body needs sodium to control the balance of fluids as well as for the proper functioning of muscles and nerves. Too much of it, however, causes water to build up inside the blood vessels, which increases blood pressure. A level of 2,300 mg per day of sodium is recommended by the DGA.

It all looks simple enough, segmented in a way we can visualize as we load up a plate at a buffet or choose what to pack for lunch on our way to work. At the same time, every publication of the DGA (at five-year intervals since 1980) elicits backlash from the industries that produce the food we eat. Food manufacturers insist that the guidelines are too restrictive and that their industries are targeted unnecessarily. A similar response comes from the medical community, often saying that the guidelines are not restrictive enough and that more emphasis needs to be placed on reduction or elimination of specific foods. Still other organizations—some representing special interests like meat and dairy producers and others touting food group-elimination diets like keto and paleo—chime in with their own objections and research they may have commissioned to "prove" their own claims.

Amid this cacophony, it can be difficult for journalists, researchers, and even peer-reviewed scientific journals to determine which points of view have merits and which are motivated by something other than the good health of the general public. Scientists face challenges of their own in attempting to understand which foods contribute to good health and which do not.

Researchers encounter ethical conundrums in using humans as test subjects, making it virtually impossible to isolate a subject's consumption of a specific food, nutrient, or ingredient to be sure that only this substance is causing a health issue. Imagine, for example, a study in which human subjects eat nothing but vegetable shortening (like Crisco or Spry) for weeks on end to see what harmful effects might emerge. Not only would the subjects exhibit health issues from consuming large amounts of trans fat, but they might very well develop diseases related to malnutrition: scurvy, rickets, anemia, beriberi, and pellagra, all of which signal vitamin deficiencies—and none of which are directly related to eating shortening. Worse, this abuse of their bodies might have the unintended consequence of jeopardizing their longer-term health.

Instead, researchers test foods first using "in vitro" studies—that is, experiments in a laboratory using microbe-sized samples in test tubes or culture dishes; and then on "mouse models," varieties of mice that share many of the same disease-causing genes that are present in humans. While thousands of studies of human diseases have begun with mouse models and have produced promising results, the studies eventually must move on to human subjects to determine if the results hold true. Designing studies that do not produce lasting harm to humans, obtaining funding for these studies, and then conducting them and reporting the results can take years, if not decades, to accomplish.

In the interim, the findings of studies on mouse models may be published in peer-reviewed journals and then reported as decisive facts by the popular media. This can turn an inconclusive study into a dictum about a specific food or nutrient long before science is ready to do so.

It is impossible, as noted earlier, to feed human beings just one food over the time it would take to produce the expected result, so human studies usually involve some kind of controlled diet that does not compromise the subjects' overall nutrition. This may mean increasing the amount of the food to be tested, while maintaining a control group that eats none of that food. For example, the test subjects may consume a helping of quinoa three times a day along with their usual meal, while the control group eats no quinoa. The researchers may then perform medical tests at regular intervals to see how the quinoa affects the subjects' health.

This may sound like solid science, but it also has its obstacles to success. Researchers usually do not have the option of sequestering the test subjects and monitoring exactly what they eat for each meal; even if the subjects were willing to make this commitment, it would be tantamount to imprisonment (and likely cost prohibitive). In most cases, subjects keep a diary of their food intake, or they are asked to recall in periodic interviews what they ate some time before. As you might guess, this can result in omissions of information and forgotten foods and meals. If the study continues for a long period of time—some of these go on for years—subjects may drop out, decide they no longer wish to participate, move away, or even die.

As if these issues did not make food studies hard enough to conduct, there are added levels of difficulty to deal with: Foods do not act in isolation in our bodies, and other things besides foods impact our health.

Nutrients often work together to produce a beneficial effect: For example, to help the body absorb calcium, vitamin D must be present in sufficient amounts. As people eat a variety of foods at the same time and each of these foods may contain a wide range of ingredients, it can be very difficult to credit one food with a specific effect on the body.

While many functions within the human body are well understood by medical science, no two people are exactly alike, and no one lives precisely the same lifestyle as anyone else. Health issues handed down genetically for many generations can make one person's body behave quite differently from another one, changing the way the body digests, absorbs, and puts a food to use. People who are more physically active and fit than others may metabolize nutrients differently from someone who leads a sedentary life that results in obesity. Chronic medical conditions, food allergies, intolerances to dairy or wheat, imbalances in all the bacteria and other microorganisms in the gut (the microbiome), the presence of autoimmune disease, and a host of other issues can make one test subject very unlike another, producing widely skewed results.

Into this din of conflicting opinions comes the consumer, trying to put healthy meals on the table for a family and confused about what "healthy" actually means. Even where the consumer buys food, new information catches the eye in the supermarket checkout line—magazine headlines that tout the latest secrets for weight loss or a way to add ten years to our lives: "Don't Eat Anything White!" "Lose Five Pounds Overnight With This One Weird Trick!" "How These Three Superfoods Will Change Your Life!" And so many others.

Are you baffled by this constant barrage of conflicting science, expert opinions, and fads? If so, it is working. Keeping consumers off-balance about the food they eat is part of the marketing plan for a wide range of weight-loss companies, food packagers, and professional associations that represent food producers and agriculture. The more they can cast doubt on the validity of basic nutritional guidelines, the more consumers will continue to question what they should and should not eat—and in this cloud of uncertainty, we are more likely to give in to our urges and eat that entire sleeve of cookies or order a bigger steak.

THE NUTRITION RESEARCH CONUNDRUM

How are consumers supposed to determine what is solid science and what is the work of a special interest group? The line between the two has become fuzzy at best. Let's take a very recent example: a study published in the *Annals of*

Internal Medicine in October 2019 by Bradley C. Johnston, epidemiologist at Dalhousie University in Canada, and a team of more than a dozen other researchers from around the world.

The study claimed that the link between red meat, heart disease, and cancer had never been proven conclusively by science, so people should not limit their consumption of beef and processed meats. This result drew immediate ire from health organizations and other scientists who had conducted their own published studies of red meat, but Johnston defended the legitimacy of the work and underscored that there were no conflicts of interest among his team—that is, no one on the research team worked for companies in the meat industry, and no industry organization had provided funds for the work.

However, the *New York Times* reported just days after the study's publication that Johnston had not disclosed that he had been a senior author on another published study several years earlier, one paid for by the International Life Sciences Institute (ILSI), "an industry trade group largely supported by agribusiness, food and pharmaceutical companies," including McDonald's, Coca-Cola, PepsiCo, and Cargill. That study attempted to discredit the science behind nutritional guidelines that advised people to eat less sugar. The *Times* quoted New York University professor Marion Nestle, who studies conflicts of interest in food research, in calling ILSI "a classic front group" for the food industry. "Even if ILSI had nothing to do with the meat paper—and there is no evidence of which I am aware that it did—the previous paper suggests that Johnston is making a career of tearing down conventional nutrition wisdom."

The *Times* sought out Christine Laine, MD, MPH, FACP, editor-in-chief of *Annals of Internal Medicine*, who pointed out that there are conflicts of interest on all sides of the meat issue, whether or not they had a hand in the study. "Many of the people who are criticizing these articles have lots of conflicts of interest they aren't talking about," she said. "They do workshops on plant-based diets, do retreats on wellness and write books on plant-based diets. There are conflicts on both sides." She added that even if there had been a direct financial relationship between the study and a special interest group, the research methodology used still would have passed muster for publication.

How, then, should the consumer process the information in the study? Is there such a thing as an unbiased study or an unbiased response to a controversial finding?

These are difficult questions to answer, but they tell us a great deal about why we see so much controversy over the foods we eat and their potential effects on our overall health. A study funded by the industry that will benefit from its results—whether the industry is food, tobacco, coal, or running shoes—may produce sound scientific results, but if these results reach publication, they almost invariably favor the industry that funded them.

"Food companies don't want to fund studies that won't help them sell products," researcher Nestle told *Vox* in 2018. "So I consider this kind of research marketing, not science."

CLAIMS VERSUS REALITY

Media reports on food studies rarely have unlimited space to provide clarifying detail, so the foreshortened summaries in newspapers, in magazines, and on websites usually reduce the message down to its tantalizing essence. This results in headlines like "11 Reasons Chocolate's Good For You," "Red Meat: It Does a Body Good!" and "Everyone Was Wrong: Saturated Fat Can Be Good For You." As the message goes out to commercial and personal websites and to blogs, it gets even more distilled and distorted, until what began as coverage of research becomes wild claims of the miraculous properties of specific foods. Suddenly chocolate has "the highest antioxidants on the planet," and red palm fruit oil will "extend the warranty of nearly every organ in your body."

Glancing at such headlines can send consumers spiraling off into unhealthy eating habits, all the while believing that they are doing the right thing for their bodies. In reality, they are simply taking the poetic exaggerations of nonexperts at their word, without reading the study—if there is one—or searching for the truth behind the claim.

These stories feed the foibles of human nature, wish fulfillment that foods that delight our senses and deliver the highest overall satisfaction will also be healthy for us. It does not take much prodding from the media before consumers embrace the supposed health benefits of chocolate instead of foods we have known to be healthy for generations: cruciferous vegetables or leafy greens, perhaps, or a cup of sliced fruit. At the same time, the lure of the single food that will reset the body's metabolic systems, clean out every toxin, and result in perfect health can spur consumers to buy products that make such claims but have no ability at all to accomplish these goals.

Studies also rarely make conclusions about the size of a serving that will have the near-magical properties of improving health. Study after study crowing over the health-giving properties of dark chocolate, for example—nearly all of which are funded by Mars, Nestle, Hershey, or Barry Callebaut, some of the largest chocolate companies in the world—tout the beneficial effects of antioxidants, but gloss over the countereffects of the sugar and fat every piece of sweetened chocolate contains. Eating lots of dark chocolate will please the palate and may have some trace of positive effect, but the caloric intake and the high doses of sugar provide exactly the opposite effect, making the confection more of a health risk than a benefit.

HEALTHY OR NOT: LABELS MAY LIE

Even foods that masquerade as healthy can pose dangerous challenges to our personal health goals. A comparison of low-fat and normal versions of packaged foods performed by researchers in 2016, for example, found that "the amount of sugar is higher in the low fat (i.e., reduced calorie, light, low fat) and non-fat than 'regular' versions of tested items." Nguyen et al. revealed what the media already believed to be true: "The food industry may have replaced fat with sugar, which may be more obesogenic even if the calories per portion are less." They found this to be true in low-fat dairy products, baked goods, meats, fish, poultry, fats, oils, and salad dressings—essentially in packaged foods in just about every category.

This may be part of the reason that the eight-year Women's Health Initiative Dietary Modification Trial, which followed the diet of nearly 49,000 women between the ages of fifty and seventy-nine from 1993 to 2001, showed that women on a low-fat diet did not lose weight, and thus did not lower their risk of breast cancer or cardiovascular disease. Many consumers find themselves in the same position, attempting to battle weight gain and avoid life-changing medical conditions by pursuing the 1977 guidelines to eat less fat, only to find the low-fat diet a complete failure for weight loss. These so-called healthy foods actually work against us, as the food industry quietly substitutes one ingredient for another in a bid to maintain delicious taste and texture, each food manufacturer's most competitive advantage.

The reaction of consumers to so much conflicting information may be to ignore the warnings they hear from the scientific community and even from their own doctors, giving them the same credence voiced by Mary Cooper, a character on the situation comedy "The Big Bang Theory": "Doctors are always changing their mind. One week bacon grease is bad for you. The next week we're not getting enough of it."

Balanced nutrition should be—and is—a fairly simple concept with some basic rules. It becomes complicated when science, marketing, and self-delusion come into play, conflicting forces that blur the lines between facts, fancy, and the quick-fix dreams of the average consumer.

RESOURCES

Belluz, Julia. "Nutrition Research Is Deeply Biased by Food Companies. A New Book Explains Why." *Vox*, Nov. 11, 2018. Accessed Jan. 13, 2020. https://www.vox.com/2018/10/31/18037756/superfoods-food-science-marion-nestle-book

Crocker, Lizzie. "The Dangers of Superfoods." *The Daily Beast*, Jul. 12, 2017. Accessed Jan. 13, 2020. https://www.thedailybeast.com/the-dangers-of-superfoods

Howard, B.V., et al. "Low-Fat Dietary Pattern and Weight Change Over 7 Years: The Women's Health Initiative Dietary Modification Trial." *JAMA*, Jan. 4, 2006, 295(1), 39–49. Accessed Jan. 13, 2020. https://www.ncbi.nlm.nih.gov/pubmed/16391215

Nestle, Marion. "Perspective: Challenges and Controversial Issues in the Dietary Guidelines for Americans, 1980–2015." *Advances in Nutrition*, Mar. 2018, 9(2), 148–150. Accessed. Jan. 12, 2020. https://academic.oup.com/advances/article/9/2/148/4969264

Nguyen, P.K.; Lin, S.; and Heidenreich, P. "A Systematic Comparison of Sugar Content in Low-Fat vs. Regular Versions of Food." *Nutrition & Diabetes*, Jan. 2016, 6(1), e193. Accessed Jan. 13, 2020. https://www.ncbi.nlm.nih.gov/pmc/articles/PMC4742721/

Parker-Pope, Tara; and O'Connor, Anashad. "Scientist Who Discredited Meat Guidelines Didn't Report Past Food Industry Ties." *The New York Times*, Oct. 4, 2019. Accessed Jan. 12, 2020. https://www.nytimes.com/2019/10/04/well/eat/scientist-who-discredited-meat-guidelines-didnt-report-past-food-industry-ties.html

U.S. Department of Agriculture. *Dietary Guidelines for Americans 2015–2020, Eighth Edition*. Office of Disease Prevention and Health Promotion. Accessed Jan. 12, 2020. https://health.gov/dietaryguidelines/2015/guidelines/

The History of Food Controversies

People have most likely debated the merits or perils of various foods since they first began to communicate with one another. We can imagine the earliest human beings arguing over the benefits of one animal's meat over another or disagreeing over which berries were tastier and which could actually kill a person with poison. The fact that some people have a gene that makes cilantro and arugula taste like soap points to a likely source of disagreement over dinner tables for centuries, but we have no way to prove this beyond common sense and conjecture.

Author Mark Kurlansky attempted to codify one of the earliest food controversies in his book *Milk! A 10,000-Year Food Fracas*. The debate centered on cheese, emerging as far back as the first written records of Greek civilization. Hippocrates, considered to this day to be the father of modern medicine, wrote in the fifth century BC about the hazards of eating cheese: "Cheese does not harm all people alike, and there are some people who can eat as much of it as they like without the slightest adverse effects. Indeed it is wonderfully nourishing food for the people with whom it agrees. But others suffer dreadfully. . .," perhaps revealing the first awareness of the symptoms of lactose intolerance.

A few centuries later, Anthimus, a Greek man of AD 500s, both agreed and disagreed with Hippocrates's early assessment. "Whoever eats baked or boiled cheese has no need of another poison," he wrote, going on to declare that cured cheese caused kidney stones, while fresh cheese was unlikely to cause any harm. His perspective echoed other writers that had set down their thoughts about cheese even earlier in the millennium, some declaring aged cheese to cause stomach agonies of many varieties, while others said that it actually assisted digestion.

Cheese is a product of milk, of course, so which milk provides the most nutritional value quickly became a side discussion. Greeks and Romans debated whether goats, sheep, or donkeys provided the most nourishing milk for babies (after mother's milk or the milk of a wet nurse) and whether or not milk would rot a human's teeth. In 1775, French doctor Alphonse Leroy delved into the causes of a high percentage of infant deaths in a hospital in Aix and concluded that the babies died from artificial feeding with animal milk, which spoiled quickly after being harvested from the animal. The discovery of pasteurization in the 1880s removed this hazard from animal milk, but the debate over the merits of breastfeeding versus artificial feeding continues today.

Meanwhile, as more people migrated from rural areas into the big cities and had to shop at markets for the food they ate, packaged products took a dark turn. Food producers from dairies to meat packagers found ways to make inferior foods look tasty and last longer on shelves, compromising health to disguise rancid, spoiled, or otherwise unpalatable milk, meat, butter, honey, syrup, and many other foods. The use of fillers and additives also extended the supply of each food, allowing packagers to make more money with less actual product. Unsuspecting consumers had no idea that they were eating brick dust instead of cinnamon, the cleaning product borax in their butter, salicylic acid in beer and wine, corn syrup instead of honey, and the poisonous preservative formaldehyde in milk and meat.

As he saw people becoming ill with strange symptoms, Dr. Harvey Washington Wiley, the chief chemist of the U.S. Department of Agriculture, determined that an investigation into the true contents of food and drink was necessary. He formed a cadre of brave volunteers that became known as The Poison Squad, young men who agreed to eat specific foods prepared for them at every meal for an extended period of time and take capsules filled with substances that were being used as preservatives and additives in many foods. Wiley then tested the men to determine the effects of these chemicals on their health.

Not surprisingly, the young men showed all kinds of symptoms of illness, especially when Wiley fed them formaldehyde. "We like to think of our great-grandparents as pink-cheeked eaters of nothing but the finest food," said Deborah Blum, author of *The Poison Squad: One Chemist's Single-Minded Crusade for Food Safety at the Turn of the Twentieth Century*, to Karl Knutson at the University of Wisconsin at Madison in 2019. "But they were eating fake, poisonous food full of really bad things."

Despite the startling results of his experiments, it took years before Wiley convinced enough people that the food industry was actively poisoning Americans. He finally managed to ensure the passage of the Pure Food and Drug Act of 1906, which required truth in food labeling and banned the nefarious practices so many food manufacturers had instituted.

In 1912, Kazimierz (Casimir) Funk, a Polish scientist, was the first to determine that foods contained "vital amines," which he later shortened to vitamins, substances that nourished the body and contributed to good health. His work led to the discovery of thiamine (vitamin B_1), riboflavin (B_2), niacin (B_3), and vitamins C and D, each of which played a role in preventing single-nutrient deficiency diseases like scurvy (vitamin C), beriberi (B_1), pellagra (B_3), rickets (D), and pernicious anemia (B_{12}). All of the major vitamins had been identified and named by the middle of the twentieth century—remarkably, just in time for the Great Depression and World War II, when governments around the world faced the very real possibility of food shortages. The German submarine warfare campaign during World War I had culminated in widespread grain shortages across Europe, as countries dependent on imports were cut off from their suppliers. Food-rationing programs had saved lives in Britain, France, and Italy, but no one wanted to see a repeat of this. The ongoing conflict with Germany throughout the 1930s indicated that another massive war was on the horizon.

The looming crisis led the League of Nations, the British Medical Association, and the U.S. government to take an important step. They each determined the recommended daily allowances (RDAs) of nutrients for the human diet as well as the caloric intake to maintain a healthy weight. In addition to vitamins, the RDAs addressed nutrients including calcium, iron, protein, and phosphorus, establishing minimums required for soldiers on the battlefield as well as for citizens at home.

The National Nutrition Conference for Defense presented these guidelines in 1941, and the *Journal of the American Medical Association* (*JAMA*) published them as well, making the information readily available to the global medical community. For the first time, food's role as the primary delivery system for nutrients became well understood by the general public as well as by the scientific and medical communities.

Which foods packed the most nutritional punch, however, and which might actually be bad for us would become the hotly contested domain of food growers, manufacturers, packagers, and their marketing departments. Manufacturers moved quickly to find ways to synthesize nutrients and fortify products with vitamins and minerals they did not normally contain. They developed processing methods that purified staples like wheat and rice, making them more shelf-stable and better able to carry synthetic nutrients. These products boosted the nutritional content of foods imported by poorer and developing countries, helping to alleviate some of their dietary issues, while giving consumers in richer countries more choices for their own families' nutrition.

After World War II and the resumption of import–export activity around the world, nutrition scientists turned their attention to noncommunicable diseases beyond those caused by vitamin deficiencies. Coronary heart disease (CHD) had become a leading cause of death in nations with an abundance of food choices, particularly in American men. This led to many studies of the role of various dietary issues in causing CHD, from fats and cholesterol to carbohydrates—including sugar, a simple carbohydrate that boosts mood and acts as a source of quick energy, but also inflames fat cells and leads to rapid weight gain. Studies also examined the role of all of the known vitamins and minerals, plant-based substances called phytosterols that we now know can help lower LDL cholesterol, and amino acids.

Research in the 1950s divided the scientific community on whether dietary fats or sugar contributed more strongly to the development of these diseases. John Yudkin's research revealed that added sugars are the primary cause of heart disease, while Ancel Keys determined that the combined total of saturated and other kinds of fat, as well as cholesterol, played an equally significant role.

As evidence mounted that sugar might be a greater heart disease trigger than fat and cholesterol, the sugar industry took steps to keep this information from coming to light.

In 2016, a research team led by Cristin E. Kearns, DDS, MBA, discovered 1,551 pages of documents in the University of Illinois Archives that included correspondence between the Sugar Research Foundation (SRF) and one of its scientific advisors, Roger Adams, written between 1959 and 1971. The team also found documents that passed between the SRF and D. Mark Hegsted, professor of nutrition at the Harvard School of Public Health, who codirected the SRF's research on CHD in 1965 and 1966.

The correspondence said that the SRF's scientific advisory board knew in 1962 that sugar could elevate cholesterol, even if people maintained a low-fat diet. By 1964, laboratories had discovered that sugar was a greater hazard to human health than other carbohydrates, replicating Yudkin's research. The SRF's vice president and director of research, John Hickson, recommended that the SRF "embark on a major program" to counteract "negative attitudes toward sugar." He suggested opinion polls, symposia to unveil fallacies behind the research, and a review of all the research to date to "see what weak points there are in the experimentation, and replicate the studies with appropriate corrections. Then we can publish the data and refute our detractors."

This started a systematic and highly effective effort to undermine findings of studies throughout the 1960s that linked sugar to CHD. The effort, known as Project 226, involved an extensive literature review titled "Dietary Fats, Carbohydrates and Atherosclerotic Disease," published in the *New England Journal of Medicine* in 1967, in which the authors did not disclose the involvement of the SRF. "The review concluded there was 'no doubt' that the only dietary intervention required to prevent CHD was to reduce dietary cholesterol and substitute polyunsaturated fat for saturated fat in the American diet," Kearns et al. wrote. "Overall, the review focused on possible bias in individual studies and types of evidence rather than on consistency across studies and the coherence of epidemiologic, experimental and mechanistic evidence."

In short, to protect market share for the sugar industry, the report led the medical community and the general public to believe that sugar played no significant role in CHD and that fat was the real culprit in clogging arteries with cholesterol. When this effort succeeded in focusing negative attention almost entirely on fat, SRF moved on to attempt to refute the fact that sugar contributed in large measure to tooth decay, though this effort did not meet with the same success.

MANY INDUSTRIES, MANY CONTROVERSIES

If this had been an isolated incident, the world's population might be far less confused over what they should and should not eat to maintain good health over a lifetime. The misleading sugar information, however, is just one of many efforts to protect the profit-making abilities of various segments of the food industries by informing the public that specific foods have properties that make them healthier than others, even when research does not bear these conclusions out.

The Sugar Association, the modern reorganization of the SRF, continued its campaign to make the public believe that not only was refined sugar a safe ingredient, but it was actually good for us. Just as the link between sugar and diabetes became well understood, a 1970s advertising campaign touted sugar as an important aid to dieting, with headlines like "Sugar can be the willpower you need to undereat." Another ad suggested that the way to "get ready for the fat time of day," referring to when people allow themselves to get very hungry, was to eat more sweets. "By snacking on something sweet shortly before mealtime, you turn your appestat down," the ad said, referring to an area of the brain that controls the appetite. "The sugar in a couple of cookies or a small dish of ice cream can turn it down almost immediately."

The scientific-sounding solution to hunger seems absurd now, but it gained some credence at the time, leading to even more perverse claims by the industry. "If sugar is so fattening," an ad dominated by an image of a bubbling cola drink over ice asked, "how come so many kids are thin?" A Milky Way candy bar commercial suggested that viewers should have a bar "whenever you're in the mood—it tastes like chocolaty candy, but it's really nourishing food! Oh, there's farm-fresh milk in a Milky Way and whipped-up egg whites, too." It ended by calling Milky Way "the Good Food Candy Bar!"

At the same time, a major shift took place in people's diets. Processed food began to overtake homemade dishes, spurred by the convenience of purchasing a packaged product and the wide availability of fast food in all but the most remote communities. The ability to feed a family in minutes and do so economically—just as the women's liberation movement saw many women reducing or rejecting their homemaker role and pursuing careers—changed the way people ate and altered the nutritional content of each meal and snack. Obesity rates began to soar, even in some of the poorest nations in the world. Hypertension, heart disease, and diabetes grew and spread throughout the world with a prevalence never seen before.

Amidst this proliferation of chronic diseases, the U.S. government presented its first *Dietary Guidelines for Americans*, a set of rules that are updated every five years to accommodate the most recent understanding of nutrition. These first guidelines seem almost quaint today with their basic advice: "Eat a variety of foods; maintain ideal weight; avoid too much fat, saturated fat and cholesterol;

eat foods with adequate starch and fiber; avoid too much sugar; avoid too much sodium; if you drink alcohol, do so in moderation."

The overly simplistic direction led the food manufacturing and packaging industry to bolster the nutritional value of its products with synthetic vitamins and minerals and to make substitutions in ingredients to reduce the amount of saturated fat. Consumers readily believed that the low-fat cookies they bought were healthier than their standard choices, never suspecting that the excellent flavor and texture they enjoyed had been created by doubling the sugar or by adding sugar products like high-fructose corn syrup. Preservatives in frozen and canned foods lengthened shelf life but had a negative effect on the food's healthfulness. Soaring sodium content provided the flavor consumers craved, but led to hypertension and kidney failure. Replacement of saturated fat with partially hydrogenated vegetable or tropical oils led to the proliferation of trans fats, which have since been found to reduce HDL (good) cholesterol while dramatically increasing LDL (bad) cholesterol—making them even worse than the fats they replaced.

In the end, many of the products advertised as healthier choices were no better for the human body than their original counterparts, and some actually did more harm than good. With new knowledge and a stronger understanding of the hazards of the modern diet, it might seem that people should be making better choices based on sound principles of nutrition and health . . . but this is not necessarily the case.

BACK-TO-NATURE DIET FADS

Some foods are healthier than others—no one would dispute this fact. The idea that some foods provide a knockout punch to disease and supply all of the nutrition the body needs in a single bite, however, is a fantasy at best. This has not stopped the marketing departments of food producers and diet purveyors from attempting to sell their products as the best alternatives for a lifetime of blissful good health.

After several decades loaded with processed foods and their additives, consumers have seen the negative effects that a steady diet of such products has had on their bodies. Moving away from bad habits and embracing a healthier, more natural diet would undoubtedly provide a better path to wellness, but consumers were left to seek a new direction on that path for themselves . . . until the next age of food marketing caught up with them.

Enter the designer diets that center on raw foods and food group elimination, touting foods served and eaten in their natural state, with anything processed (or, in some cases, anything cooked) treated as evil—unless, of course, it has the diet's brand name on it. Atkins, keto, paleo, and South Beach diets all eliminate carbohydrates except for small portions of fruit and vegetables, but instead of centering on lean proteins as healthier choices, they encourage a significant increase in saturated fat—a risky proposition because of its well-known link to heart disease. Some of these diets also feature packaged products that bear the diet's logo, from snacks to full meals, each with its nontrivial price tag. These diets have been known to exacerbate liver and kidney disease by overwhelming these organs with hard-to-digest fats, while leading to nutrient deficiencies from reductions in fruit, vegetables, and grains.

"Power foods" emerged as well, grouping specific fruits, vegetables, grains, and nuts with manufactured products like fortified bottled water and a tangy yogurt-based drink called kombucha. Some foods made "top 10" lists, signifying them as the healthiest things a person can eat or foods touted to aid in weight loss, increase energy, or even reverse heart disease and diabetes.

Can there be truth to these claims that all the vitamins, minerals, and other nutrients we need have been right here under our noses all along—and all we need to do is eat these five or ten or twelve amazing things and forsake everything else? How can we be sure that following the advice of the latest studies and headlines will be good for us—or at least not bad for us?

This book endeavors to break down these and many other food controversies to better understand which messages have a basis in fact and which are nothing more than marketing hype. While this book does not attempt to bring any of these disputed issues to an absolute conclusion, the analysis may help readers recognize a dubious claim and apply a critical eye and ear to the next story they may want to believe, but that simply doesn't carry that ring of truth.

RESOURCES

"Antioxidants and Cancer Prevention." National Cancer Institute. Accessed Jan. 16, 2020. https://www.cancer.gov/about-cancer/causes-prevention/risk/diet/antioxidants-fact-sheet

Blum, Deborah. *The Poison Squad: One Chemist's Single-Minded Crusade for Food Safety at the Turn of the Twentieth Century*. New York: Penguin Random House, 2019.

Garber, Megan. "If Sugar Is Fattening, How Come So Many Kids Are Thin?" *The Atlantic*, June 19, 2015. Accessed Jan. 16, 2020. https://www.theatlantic.com/entertainment/archive/2015/06/if-sugar-is-fattening-how-come-so-many-kids-are-thin/396380/

Kearns, Cristin E.; Schmidt, Laura A.; and Glantz, Stanton A. "Sugar Industry and Coronary Heart Disease Research: A Historical Analysis of Internal Industry Documents." *JAMA Internal Medicine*, Oct. 3, 2018. Accessed Jan. 16, 2020. https://www.ncbi.nlm.nih.gov/pmc/articles/PMC5099084/

Knutson, Karl. "Go Big Read Book 'The Poison Squad' Offers Food for Thought." *W News*, University of Wisconsin-Madison, Oct. 9, 2019. Accessed Mar. 12, 2020. https://news.wisc.edu/go-big-read-book-the-poison-squad-offers-food-for-thought/

Kurlansky, Mark. *Milk! A 10,000-Year Food Fracas*. New York: Bloomsbury Publishing, 2019.

Mozaffarian, Dariush, et al. "History of Modern Nutrition Science—Implications for Current Research, Dietary Guidelines, and Food Policy." *BMJ*, June 13, 2018, 261(2392). https://www.bmj.com/content/361/bmj.k2392

"Nutrition and Your Health: Dietary Guidelines for Americans." U.S. Department of Agriculture, 1980. Accessed Jan. 16, 2020. https://health.gov/dietaryguidelines/1980thin.pdf?_ga=2.55721323.1311854758.1579207439-1493036851.1578858966

O'Connor, Anahad. "How the Sugar Industry Shifted Blame to Fat." *The New York Times*, Sept. 12, 2016. Accessed Jan. 16, 2020. https://www.nytimes.com/2016/09/13/well/eat/how-the-sugar-industry-shifted-blame-to-fat.html

"Should You Try the Keto Diet?" Harvard Health Publishing, Harvard Medical School, Dec. 12, 2019. Accessed Jan. 27, 2020. https://www.health.harvard.edu/staying-healthy/should-you-try-the-keto-diet

How to Evaluate Nutrition Research and Health Claims

New information about nutrition makes headlines almost every day, whether it is found in a national newspaper, on a respected news website, in a medical journal, or on a blog of uneven reputation. It can be exceedingly difficult for the average consumer to understand if we should take the information with a grain of salt or if we should embrace it as the new normal.

Which information is reliable, and which is a carefully veiled marketing message from a food company? How can we tell credible science from slick packaging? Most people struggle to tell the difference, while others simply accept anything they see in the media as established fact.

"Nutrition research is complex, and is often oversimplified by the media," said an article from the Harvard T.H. Chan School of Public Health. "Writers may report on a single preliminary study that is unverified by additional research, or highlight a study because it contradicts current health recommendations—the goal being an attention-grabbing headline."

Generally, each new scientific study is another step toward gaining an understanding of how the body works and how nutrients affect it, but no single study is the absolute final word on science. Research continues at universities and other institutions around the globe on a daily basis, with each new finding providing a small advancement or a small setback in our knowledge. We as consumers tend to seek the once-and-for-all truth about what we should be eating and how much of it we should eat to achieve a desired result, but there may never be a single answer to these questions—and the answer may be different from one individual to the next.

Different kinds of studies may test the same hypothesis and yield different results. This may be because one study's methodology is more solid and reliable than another or because one study involved thousands of cases, while another used a very small sample group. In some cases, the contradictory studies are equally credible, but the research arrived at different conclusions—and this leads to more questions and more research to understand why.

News headlines meant to increase viewership or grab a reader's attention can color our judgment as well. "Fruits and Vegetables Are Trying to Kill You," an article in the ezine *Nautilus* proclaims, when the text of the article discusses how plant-based eating improves health by providing antioxidants that neutralize free radicals in the body. "Chocolate Can Save Your Life," a headline in the *Independent*, a newspaper in the United Kingdom, told its readers, espousing the effects of antioxidants and the limited effect those in chocolate might have in preventing cancer. The website for People for the Ethical Treatment of Animals (PETA) carries this story: "Here's Why Eating Fish Is Actually Really Bad For You," portraying all fish as laden with mercury and PCBs (banned since 1977) and therefore virtually poisonous. All of these stories have their basis in research, but their meaning has been distorted to lure readers—and in at least one case, to advance a special interest agenda.

"What's missing from the increasingly fast-paced media world is context," Harvard's T.H. Chan School tells us. "Diet stories in the news often provide little information about how the newly reported results fit in with existing evidence on the topic, which may result in exaggerating the new study's importance."

Before taking any news report about a research study at face value, consumers can develop their own ability to read and listen critically and to determine if the study has merit, if it is a shill for a corporation or industry's interests, if it is simply nonsense, or if they should seek additional information before accepting its findings. Here are some guidelines to follow to help you become a more critical reader of scientific research in all its forms.

1. **What kind of study is this**? There are many kinds of studies, and some are much more likely to produce an accurate result than others.
   a. *Meta-analysis* combines data from a number of already completed studies to arrive at a conclusion. This method can strengthen the validity of the results because there are more subjects involved, increasing the study's diversity and delivering a more statistically significant result.
   b. *Systematic review.* This process, also known as a literature review, is usually conducted by a panel of researchers who review all of the studies on a specific topic and compile a report for publication. The report summarizes the findings of each study and draws one or more conclusions about the data overall. Some such reviews do not take into account the widely varying methods used by the many studies, which may have led to very different results. Systematic reviews should screen out studies that are outliers because of their research methods or a major difference in focus, using only the studies that are relevant to the specific question asked by the review.
   c. *Randomized controlled trial.* The most credible and often the costliest of the many study designs, the randomized trial assigns subjects randomly to either an experimental group or a control group. The experimental group tests whatever the variable

is—a new drug, a specific diet, a practice like exercise or therapy—while the control group does something else or does nothing at all. This allows the researchers to determine if the specific variable has an effect on the experimental group, in comparison to those who did not have that variable. The clear identification of the participants, the ability to screen out other variables, and the randomization all make this the most reliable form of research.

d. *Cohort study*. Sometimes short term and sometimes continuing for years or decades, the cohort study follows a specific group to determine its risk factors for a disease, a condition, or another result. People in the study usually share similar characteristics (e.g., women in their twenties who all weigh between 120 and 140 pounds). The study introduces a variable—like adding an avocado per week to their diet for a year—which in turn becomes a risk factor with a potential outcome. The researchers then monitor the cohort's compliance with the study variable, collect data, and determine the effect of the variable at the end of the study. There can be drawbacks to cohort studies, however: They may take place in a contained geographic area where other variables can interfere with the outcome or the cohort itself may not be random enough to produce a valid result.

e. *Case control study*. Here no actual variables are tested. The study is based on observation of subjects selected because they already have a specific disease, condition, or lifestyle. The study examines the subjects' past behavior after the fact to determine if the behavior affects the disease or condition. Because this kind of study attempts to trace the cause after the effect is known, it must rely on the subject's recollection of things he or she did days, months, or years before. The result may be biased by coincidences, triggering the fallacy *post hoc ergo propter hoc*—which translates to "after that, therefore because of that." For example, a study may look at people with cancer to determine how much red meat they ate before their diagnosis. The results would rely on people's memory of how often they ate burgers or steak over the course of years, without taking into account other factors like a genetic predisposition to cancer, exposure to environmental factors, and other potential causes of their condition.

f. *Case report*. Not strictly a study, a case report is an article that describes a specific incident or subject, usually one that is an outlier or is otherwise unique. It may, for example, examine the case of a woman who eats avocados every day and who also develops rosacea, a rosy skin condition on her face. These two things may or may not have anything to do with one another, but the case report may work to draw parallels between these two disparate things. If other scientists or doctors have observed the same variables, they may read the case report in a journal and contact the scientist who wrote the paper, which may lead to a case control study and, eventually, a randomized trial.

2. **How many studies are involved?** A single study rarely provides all the information the scientific community needs to declare its results to be unshakingly valid. This is especially true if the study is actually a case report about one individual or a case control study that attempts to piece together behavior from memories. These studies may indicate the need for additional research, but they cannot be taken as the final word.

3. **Who paid for the study?** Most peer-reviewed journals require researchers to disclose the funders of their studies, which will be either mentioned in the study abstract or listed at the end of the publication. Studies may be highly suspect if they provide these

funders with the scientific data they need to declare their products to be miraculously healthy. This may be the most telling aspect of whether you as a consumer should take the study's findings to heart. As we have seen earlier in this book and will see again going forward, food industry executives have a great deal invested in keeping their products on the market, and some will pay to boost their claims of healthiness and bury the truth about the potential negative effects of their own products. This is the very definition of conflict of interest in food science. Such studies can certainly produce plausible results if the methodology is sound and if the food industry association remained hands-off, providing the funding but allowing the researchers to come to data-driven conclusions on their own. It is up to the peers who review these studies before publication to determine the level of involvement the funders had and if they interfered in the results in any way. Publication does not automatically mean that there is no bias, but it can be a good indicator that the review committee found the research to be credible.

4. **Are the subjects humans or animals**? Dietary studies may not always involve human subjects. Animal studies often come before human studies, but their results may not translate to humans and should not be taken as the final word on the health benefits of a specific food, diet, medication, therapy, or any other practice. Ninety-five percent of studies use mice or rats, in part because their genetic and biological characteristics are remarkably similar to humans—and scientists can breed "transgenic" mice with genes that are very like the ones that cause diseases in people. Not every result achieved in rodents can be duplicated in a human being, however; researchers will move on to studies with humans if their results are exciting enough to bring them more funding.
5. **How big a study is it?** A study involving just a few subjects may be more anecdotal than scientific, as the sample may not be statistically significant. Larger studies usually provide more dependable results, but they can be very costly to develop and manage, making it difficult for a university or independent research organization to acquire funding until they can point to significant results from a smaller study.
6. **What protocols are in place?** Be wary of so-called research that takes place outside of a well-controlled scientific setting. People who are not university researchers can have good ideas, of course, but slapdash studies do not yield reliable results, no matter how passionate the researcher may be. (One study discussed in this book took place in the researcher's home kitchen and does not pass for scientific rigor.)

Nutrition science continues to evolve, so what we believed to be fundamentally sound one day may be flipped on its head by new research the next. We learned in the 1970s, for example, that eating eggs increases the body's cholesterol level, which can lead to heart disease. Equally credible research in 2015 then told us that eggs' nutritional content outweighs their negative effects, allowing them to re-enter the *Dietary Guidelines for Americans* in 2015 as a good source of protein. In 2019, however, research published in *JAMA* found a direct association between consuming one and a half eggs daily and development of heart disease, even leading to early death.

Were we bamboozled by bad information back in the twentieth century? Or has science improved and moved on, giving us better data? The clear answer is the latter one: Science keeps improving, as jarring as it may be to have our "common knowledge" ripped away from us repeatedly over time. It is up to us as consumers of information to learn to distinguish between good science and marketing schemes, between solid research and self-interest, and among too-good-to-be-true claims, scare tactics, and provable facts.

RESOURCES

"Diet In the News—What to Believe?" Harvard T.H. Chan School of Public Health. Accessed Jan. 17, 2020. https://www.hsph.harvard.edu/nutritionsource/media/

Melina, Remy. "Why Do Medical Researchers Use Mice?" LiveScience, Nov. 16, 2010. Accessed Jan. 19, 2020. https://www.livescience.com/32860-why-do-medical-researchers-use-mice.html

Nagler, Rebecca. "Adverse Outcomes Associated with Media Exposure to Contradictory Nutrition Messages." *Journal of Health Communication*, 2014, 19(1), 24–40. Accessed Jan. 17, 2020. https://www.ncbi.nlm.nih.gov/pmc/articles/PMC4353569/

Powell, Denise. "Health Effects of Eggs: Where Do We Stand?" *CNN*, Mar. 27, 2019. Accessed Jan. 17, 2020. https://www.cnn.com/2019/03/27/health/eggs-good-or-bad-where-do-we-stand/index.html

"Study Design 101." Himmelfarb Health Sciences Library. Accessed Jan. 17, 2020. https://himmelfarb.gwu.edu/tutorials/studydesign101/

Foods and Ingredients

Artificial Flavorings

WHAT ARE THEY?

All matter in the universe is composed of chemicals—the air we breathe, the clothes we wear, the chair you're sitting in now, the scenery or objects around you, and the foods we eat. If you can see any object and touch it, taste it, or smell it, you can be certain that it is made of chemicals.

Our bodies contain all kinds of chemicals that make up our organs, bones, and even our thought processes. Oxygen, nitrogen, carbon dioxide, salt, water, blood, urine, bile, serotonin, dopamine, all kinds of electrolytes, and all of the other substances that make our bodies function are vital chemicals, required for life to exist.

The aroma and flavor of all foods come from each food's chemical makeup and its ability to activate the senses of both smell and taste. Some are volatile chemicals that evaporate and enter our nostrils, allowing us to inhale the food's scent. The sense of smell plays an important role in aiding the sense of taste—in fact, taste is our most limited sense, with taste buds in the tongue acting on just four components in food: sweet, salty, sour, and bitter (though there has been considerable discussion about "umami," a Japanese word for the taste of meaty foods, that also seems to activate selected taste buds). The combination of the senses of smell and taste creates flavor, the more intense experience of a food beyond the basics the tongue can discern on its own.

For more than a century, the food industry has researched and determined ways to increase the tastiness in foods, making the flavor as enticing as possible to keep consumers coming back for more. Artificial flavorings play a significant role in this, by distilling a flavor down to its essence—the chemicals known as esters, which provoke the strongest recognition by the taste buds—and increasing the use of this core flavor component in a specific food. Some of these chemicals occur naturally, while others can be created in laboratories from combinations of synthetic chemicals.

The U.S. FDA's Code of Federal Regulations, Title 21, Chapter 1, defines an artificial flavoring as "any substance, the function of which is to impart flavor, which is not derived from a spice, fruit or fruit juice, vegetable or vegetable juice, edible yeast, herb, bark, bud, root, leaf or similar plant material, meat, fish, poultry, eggs, dairy products, or fermentation products thereof." In other words, any flavoring that does not come from the natural source of that flavor is considered artificial. Both artificial and natural flavors may be created in laboratories, but the ingredients used to create the flavor may come from natural sources like those listed by the FDA or from both natural and artificial sources. Few flavorings can succeed if they have none of the original food's natural essence: A strawberry-flavored hard candy, for example, must derive its flavor from the essence of a strawberry, at least in part.

"There is little substantive difference in the chemical compositions of natural and artificial flavorings," writes Gary Reineccius, a professor of food science at the University of Minnesota.

> They are both made in a laboratory by a trained professional, a "flavorist," who blends appropriate chemicals together in the right proportions. The flavorist uses "natural" chemicals to make natural flavorings and "synthetic" chemicals to make artificial flavorings. The flavorist creating an artificial flavoring must use the *same* chemicals in his formulation as would be used to make a natural flavoring, however. Otherwise, the flavoring will not have the desired flavor. The distinction in flavorings—natural versus artificial—comes from the *source* of these identical chemicals and may be likened to saying that an apple sold in a gas station is artificial and one sold from a fruit stand is natural.
>
> (Reineccius, 2002)

The difference, then, comes from where the chemical itself originates. Collection of some flavors from their sources in nature can be costly and, in the case of some exotic flavors, destructive to fragile plants or crops that may be difficult to cultivate and maintain. Researchers have found ways to synthesize the same ester in a laboratory, often duplicating the plant's ester exactly using the same chemical elements to create the compound. The flavor may be identical, but the compound originated in a lab, so the FDA defines it as artificial.

CURRENT CONSUMPTION STATISTICS AND TRENDS

Estimates indicate that 90 percent of processed foods—the packaged products we purchase in grocery stores—contain artificial flavorings, making them absolutely pervasive in our food supply.

NUTRITIONAL INFORMATION

Generally, artificial flavors have little to no nutritional value. They serve the purpose of making food taste good, but they do not add vitamin or mineral content.

HISTORY

Spices, herbs, and other flavorings have been part of the human consciousness for thousands of years, but the ability to create artificial flavors came about in the 1800s, when businesses in Germany and Switzerland found ways to extract naturally occurring flavors from plants. They began to export essential oils, which contained pure esters, as well as flavor extracts that used alcohol or other carriers to increase the volume of a concentrated flavor.

By the turn of the twentieth century, food manufacturers and packagers began to spring up in the United States at a great rate, so some enterprising Americans who had imported German and Swiss flavor products—mostly in New Jersey—opened their own laboratories. As there has never been a shortage in demand for flavors, these labs continue to turn out new, interesting products to enhance the taste of processed foods. Today artificial flavors are used in thousands of packaged foods, with the market for lightly flavored sparkling waters one of the newest popular uses for these chemical compounds.

In 1938, after 100 people died when they took a popular drug containing a new, untested additive called sulfanilamide, Congress passed the Federal Food, Drug, and Cosmetic Act, requiring that all substances used in food and drugs be categorized and assessed for safety—and over the years, this law has been amended many times to make its enforcement less unwieldy. One such change was the 1958 Food Additives Amendment, which required that all food additives be approved as safe before coming to market. (More on how this works in "The Controversy" section.)

THE CONTROVERSY

Food labels tell consumers when artificial flavors have been used to create the products they buy, so it's no secret that most packaged products contain flavors synthesized in a laboratory. It is important to read beyond the ingredients to see how the manufacturer positions and modifies the product name and description, as this tells consumers a great deal about whether the product comes by its flavors naturally or via the lab. "Blueberry yogurt" may be flavored with actual blueberries, for example, while "blueberry-flavored yogurt" probably contains a substance that includes a synthesized blueberry flavor.

The larger questions, however, are whether any of these flavorings are somehow harmful to consumers or whether food manufacturers are using these flavors to trick the human body into craving more, thus luring consumers to want more of a specific cookie, candy, or chip.

As far back as 1959, the Flavor and Extract Manufacturers Association of the United States (FEMA) saw the need to establish a program through which professionals in the flavoring industry could determine the safety of the many artificial flavors proposed for use in food products. As such a testing operation had never existed before, an expert panel came together in 1960 to create a standardized program for assessing the safety of these substances, "including the use of metabolic studies and structural relationships that had not previously been applied in a significant manner to food ingredients before the Panel did so in the 1960s," according to FEMA's website. As a result of this rigorous review, artificial flavorings earned the status "Generally Regarded as Safe" (GRAS). This status means that a food ingredient has met the four criteria stated by FEMA (https://www.femaflavor.org/gras):

1. General recognition of safety by qualified experts.
2. The experts must be qualified via training and experience to evaluate the substance.
3. The experts must base their determination of safety on scientific procedures or on common use in food prior to 1958, when the program began.
4. The GRAS determination must take into account the conditions of intended use: for example, its function as a flavoring in food.

A food manufacturer cannot simply say that this review took place and the food is safe; it must be able to provide documentation for review by the FDA or other interested parties.

In addition, the Joint Expert Committee on Food Additives (JECFA) also evaluates artificial flavors for their safety to humans. This international scientific committee is overseen by the Food and Agricultural Organization of the United Nations and the World Health Organization.

The results of all of these assessments are contained in a massive database on the FDA's website, titled "Substances Added to Food," and found at https://www.accessdata.fda.gov/scripts/fdcc/?set=FoodSubstances. Any consumer can search this database and click on the name of an ingredient to see its chemical composition and its purpose in food and then click on the substance's GRAS numerical code to see the complete scientific analysis by FEMA committee or JECFA.

Seven naturally occurring chemicals used as artificial flavors have been found to cause cancer in laboratory animals when consumed in large amounts. These were banned by the FDA in 2018 and are no longer in use as food additives in the United States, though some are still used to add scent to cosmetics and other products. They include benzophenone, which produces the floral smell in grapes and other fruits; ethyl acrylate, a fruity flavor found in pineapple; methyl eugenol, a spicy-tasting compound found in some essential oils; myrcene, which gives allspice its spicy pungency; pulegone, the minty compound found in peppermint and spearmint plants, orange mint, catnip, blackcurrant, and pennyroyal; pyridine, a sour flavor with a fishy smell, originally isolated in crude coal tar; and styrene, usually synthesized from plants in the *Styrax* genus, which also provides the naturally sweet taste in some fruits, vegetables, and nuts.

The flavor industry, then, has worked to protect the public from substances that may indeed be harmful and inappropriate for human consumption. This has not stopped many organizations and people with their own agendas from working to demonize artificial flavors, however. NaturesHappiness.com (http://blogs.natureshappiness.com/artificial-flavors-side-effects/), for example, insists that "studies suggest that the side effects of artificial flavorings range from nervous system depression, dizziness, chest pain, headaches, fatigue, allergies, brain damage, seizures, and nausea. Some of the most popular flavorings can also cause genetic defects, tumors and bladder cancer to name a few." The blog's agenda, of course, is to sell "natural" nutritional supplements, and the sources it provides for its information are within its own website. To be fair, some of the artificial flavors approved as GRAS have been found to be carcinogens at very high doses, but much higher than the amount a human being would consume. FEMA has considered such cases and determined that the substance is being used at a safe level, saying, "The results from animal studies are not relevant to human safety."

John Bloom, PhD, writing for the American Council on Science and Health, sums up this issue with clarity:

> When bad science is promoted, it is reasonable to assume that there are economic benefits to be gained by those who are behind the scare-mongering. . . . Thanks to marketing campaigns that are anti-science at their core, the American public has been conditioned to equate artificial flavoring with harmful chemicals. Consumers are bombarded by terms such as "organic," "natural," and "synthetic" wherever they shop, without having anything close to a clear definition of what each term means.

So these flavorings may be generally regarded as safe, but are they addictive? It is difficult to find a credible source on the subject, though there are thousands of blogs and websites written by nonscientists who decry these substances and their use to manipulate the taste buds.

Harvard University's website contains an essay by PhD candidate C. Rose Kennedy of the Department of Chemistry and Chemical Biology, in which she notes,

> Flavors are used to amplify or modulate the sensory experience associated with existing qualities of a product. Furthermore, they may also be used to make healthy yet bland options (like those lacking an excess of sugar or trans-fat) more appealing. For example, flavor agents may make reduced-fat foods seem rich and creamy, or add salty zest to low-sodium products.

Artificial flavors contain no components that form a physical addiction, but they may promote cravings for more of the flavored food. A number of professional flavorists quoted in media reports ranging from the *New York Times* to the CBS news show *60 Minutes* describe an intention to create a powerful burst of flavor that quickly fades, making the consumer want more. Artificial flavors may also be used to intensify a flavor beyond its natural counterpart—such as a robust, sweet flavor of a raspberry candy versus the taste of an actual raspberry. Some bloggers suggest that this creates an unrealistic expectation of the flavor of real fruit in children who eat candy, but this may bring up a larger question of the availability of fresh fruit to a child—or of a parent's own choices—rather than an intentional deception by the candy maker.

FURTHER READINGS

"About FEMA GRAS Program." Flavor & Extract Manufacturers Association, 2018. Accessed July 24, 2019. https://www.femaflavor.org/gras

"Benzophenone." Chemical safetyfacts.org. Accessed July 24, 2019. https://www.chemical safetyfacts.org/benzophenone/

Bloom, Josh. "Natural and Artificial Flavors: What's the Difference?" American Council on Science and Health, New York, 2017, 29. Accessed July 24, 2019. https://www.acsh .org/sites/default/files/Natural-and-Artificial-Flavors-What-s-the-Difference.pdf

"CFR: Code of Federal Regulations, Title 21, Sec. 101.22." U.S. Food and Drug Administration, revised Apr. 1, 2018. Accessed July 17, 2019. https://www.accessdata.fda.gov /scripts/cdrh/cfdocs/cfcfr/cfrsearch.cfm?fr=101.22

"Chemical Cuisine." Center for Science in the Public Interest. Accessed July 24, 2019. https://cspinet.org/eating-healthy/chemical-cuisine#banned

"Ethyl acrylate." PubChem, U.S. National Library of Medicine, National Institutes of Health. Accessed July 24, 2019. https://pubchem.ncbi.nlm.nih.gov/compound/Ethyl -acrylate

Kennedy, C. Rose. "The Flavor Rundown: Natural vs. Artificial Flavors." Science in the News, Harvard University Graduate School of Arts and Sciences, Sept. 21, 2015. Accessed July 24, 2019. http://sitn.hms.harvard.edu/flash/2015/the-flavor-rundown -natural-vs-artificial-flavors/

"Methyleugenol." PubChem, U.S. National Library of Medicine, National Institutes of Health. Accessed July 24, 2019. https://pubchem.ncbi.nlm.nih.gov/compound/7127

"Myrcene." PubChem, U.S. National Library of Medicine, National Institutes of Health. Accessed July 24, 2019. https://pubchem.ncbi.nlm.nih.gov/compound/31253

"Pulegone." PubChem, U.S. National Library of Medicine, National Institutes of Health. Accessed July 24, 2019. https://pubchem.ncbi.nlm.nih.gov/compound/442495

"Pyridine." PubChem, U.S. National Library of Medicine, National Institutes of Health. Accessed July 24, 2019. https://pubchem.ncbi.nlm.nih.gov/compound/1049

Reineccius, Gary. "What Is the Difference Between Artificial and Natural Flavors?" *Scientific American*, July 29, 2002. Accessed July 17, 2019. https://www.scientificamerican .com/article/what-is-the-difference-be-2002-07-29/

Stokes, Abbey. "Understanding How Natural and Artificial Flavors Impact Food Product Naming." Merieux NutriSciences, May 31, 2018. Accessed July 17, 2019. http://foodsafety.merieuxnutrisciences.com/2018/05/31/understanding-how-natural -artificial-flavors-impact-food-product-naming/

"Styrene." PubChem, U.S. National Library of Medicine, National Institutes of Health. Accessed July 24, 2019. https://pubchem.ncbi.nlm.nih.gov/compound/7501

"Substances Added to Food." U.S. Food and Drug Administration, last updated Apr. 22, 2019. Accessed July 24, 2019. https://www.accessdata.fda.gov/scripts/fdcc/?set=Food Substances

Wendee, Nicole. "Secret Ingredients: Who Knows What's in Your Food?" *Environmental Health Perspectives*, Apr. 2013, 121(4), a126–a133. Accessed July 24, 2019. https:// www.ncbi.nlm.nih.gov/pmc/articles/PMC3620743/

Artificial Food Colors

WHAT ARE THEY?

Artificial food colors (AFCs), also known as food dyes, are colors made from chemicals or from natural substances and are used to improve or enhance the appearance of foods to make them more appetizing. A wide variety of substances have been used to make these dyes, but today's dyes are largely petroleum based. Only nine AFCs are currently approved as safe by the U.S. FDA for use in food. Many others have turned out to be toxic and have been banned.

Each dye is approved for use with a specific food or foods; to expand to additional uses, the dye must be reapproved by the FDA as an additive for that food. Red No. 40, for example, can be used in cereals, gelatins, dairy products, puddings, beverages, and confections, while Orange B has only received approval for use in hot dog and sausage casings. The FDA tests and certifies each individual batch of approved food color for purity and safety before it can be used in any foods.

CURRENT CONSUMPTION STATISTICS AND TRENDS

Red Dye 40 (Allura Red), Yellow No. 5 (Tartrazine), and Yellow No. 6 (Sunset Yellow) make up 90 percent of the food dyes used in the United States. Six other dyes, including additional shades of red, yellow, orange, green, and blue, complete the fairly narrow assortment of dyes used in packaged products. Breakfast cereals, vitamin pills, candy, beverages, snacks, and other edibles often contain these dyes, especially products with children as their primary targets. They are also used to "correct" the colors of natural products, such as fruit, cheese, and packaged meat.

Ameena Batada at the University of North Carolina and Michael F. Jacobson at the Center for Science in the Public Interest completed a study in 2014 in which they examined 810 products purchased in a North Carolina grocery store. All of the products they chose were marketed heavily to children. The researchers found that 350 of these products contained artificial food dyes: Nearly 30 percent had Red 40; 24.2 percent contained Blue 1; 20.5 percent contained Yellow 5; and 19.5 percent used Yellow 6. Candy had the highest percentage of food dyes (96.3 percent), while 94 percent of fruit-flavored snacks were artificially colored. Not surprisingly, 89.7 percent of drink mix powders were colored with food dyes.

In 2014, a study by Laura Stevens et al. determined that children, on average, consume 100–200 mg of AFCs per day.

NUTRITIONAL INFORMATION

AFCs provide no vitamins, minerals, or other nutritional value to the foods they color. They add no calories to food.

HISTORY

The first records of coloring foods with natural dyes came from Egypt in 1500 BC, but controversy didn't emerge in the coloring process until the late 1200s, under England's King Edward I. Wealthy people of the time preferred white flour and white bread to the darker breads made for peasants, but the common people became dissatisfied with their lower-class bread and demanded a white bread alternative that they could afford. Bakeries complied by using inexpensive alternative ingredients to lighten the bread—like lime and chalk instead of white flour. This, of course, made the bread less palatable and made those who ate it quite ill. The London government took action, making the first known law against food adulteration:

> If any default shall be found in the bread of a baker in the city, the first, time, let him be drawn upon a hurdle from the Guildhall to his own house through the great street where there be most people assembled, and through the streets which are most dirty, with the faulty loof [*sic*] hanging from his neck.

A second offense got the baker a session of verbal and physical abuse on the pillory, and if, after all of this punishment, the baker still persisted in coloring bread with dangerous substances, he or she would be forbidden from baking forever.

Additional laws came to pass over the next several hundred years, with a French bill forbidding the coloring of butter in 1396 and another in 1574 that prohibited bakers from using food dyes to color pastries so they looked as if eggs were used in their preparation.

The first mass-market exposure of the dangers of many substances used to color food came in 1820, with the publication of *A Treatise on Adulterations of Food and Culinary Poisons*, by Friedrich Accum, an English chemist. Among the many abuses he detailed, Accum noted that pickles often were colored with copper so they would appear bright green; bakers continued to color bread white, but now used metallic salts also used in styptic pencils to stanch bleeding; and candy manufacturers used mercury, lead, and dyes that contained copper and even arsenic to achieve the bright colors that attracted children to buy them.

In 1856, Sir William Henry Perkin of England used aniline, an organic compound synthesized from coal tar, to develop new food dyes that were somewhat safer than the dyes made from metal salts. Coal-tar dyes produced brighter colors, but required the use of a tiny fraction of the amount of more harmful food dyes to achieve the desired color. Denmark and Germany both passed laws in the 1850s to ban the use of colors that contained harmful chemicals. England finally followed suit in 1860 with the Food Adulteration Act, but real change did not come until the Sale of Food and Drugs Act of 1875, which made the use of harmful chemicals in food a criminal offense.

Laws in the United States did not catch up with the toxic colorants issue for some time. The government began looking into the problem in 1881, but it took until the Pure Food and Drug Act of 1906, the first consumer protection law, for

Congress to ban the use of colored metal salts and other harmful substances in food. This law's requirements only covered food and drugs sold across state lines, however, and it focused primarily on preservatives and on truth in food labeling.

Before the law, one food coloring battle became legendary in the history of additives. Margarine entered the market in the late 1800s, spurring the dairy industry to look for ways to keep this butter replacement out of stores or at least to make it unappetizing to consumers. Claims by a dairy publicity campaign that margarine actually carried cancer "germs" and was made from soap, paint, animal intestines, and even old boots made a definite impression on consumers, leading seven states to ban margarine altogether. The Supreme Court overturned these laws as restraint of trade, so the dairy industry tried another tack: They attacked margarine's color, saying that white margarine could not possibly compete with the naturally hued golden-yellow butter. States banned the manufacture of margarine that was artificially colored yellow, saying that the color only served to deceive the public into thinking it was really butter. Eventually Congress took a nationwide step, levying a margarine tax and licensing fee that made yellow margarine more expensive to consumers than real butter.

In the decades-long battle that ensued, margarine manufacturers tried to get around the tax by actually selling white margarine with packets of yellow dye enclosed, so consumers could mix in the color themselves. Realizing the ludicrousness of this, Congress finally repealed its tax in 1950 and included specific, less restrictive rules about margarine color in the Federal Food, Drug, and Cosmetic Act in the same year. In 1967, the last law against coloring margarine—not surprisingly, in the dairy state of Wisconsin—was finally repealed.

The next food dye scandal came in the 1960s, when studies began to indicate that red dye 2 might be carcinogenic. The FDA placed the dye on its provisional list until the science could be sorted out, but additional studies yielded inconsistent results, including a large Russian effort that may not even have tested the right dye. Finally, the FDA conducted its own study, which turned out to be even less dependable than the Russian one—in fact, it earned the permanent moniker "the botched FDA experiment." Whether the dye actually causes more cancerous tumors in rats, and whether this result translates to human beings, has never been proven conclusively. Amidst considerable controversy, however, the FDA took the step to delist red dye 2 from its approved AFCs in 1976, putting an end to the discussion.

Today's AFC formulations use petroleum instead of coal, assuaging some fears that the dyes were actively toxic. Not all manufacturers rely on chemicals to color their products, however. Some have turned to natural food coloring agents, including carotenoids (the bright orange of carrots), chlorophyll (which gives all green plants their color), anthocyanin (the blue and purple of blueberries, grapes, and cranberries), turmeric (the yellow of mustards), and cochineal (a brilliant red derived from insects). These dyes are costly to produce, however, as they require growing and harvesting plants in season and considerable effort to process the material and extract the colors. They also spoil quickly, making their shelf life very short for the amount of trouble they are to make. Worse, cochineal dye triggers a severe allergic reaction in some people, including anaphylactic shock.

Some natural colors may actually have nutritive value, however, making them preferable as the market demands that food be free of artificial additives and that food producers maximize the health benefits of their products.

THE CONTROVERSY

The question of whether AFCs and other food additives have an effect on attention-deficit/hyperactivity disorder (ADHD)—or even cause the disorder—has kept researchers busy for generations dating back to the 1920s. The first to draw a direct connection between ADHD and AFCs was pediatric allergist Benjamin Feingold, who reported in 1973 that his research showed a link between hyperactivity and an assortment of food additives, including salicylates, artificial colors, artificial flavors, and preservatives BHA and BHT. He designed a diet free of these added chemicals, which became known as the Kaiser Permanante diet and later as the Feingold diet. His two books, *Why Your Child Is Hyperactive* and *The Feingold Cookbook for Hyperactive Children*, became national bestsellers . . . but by 1983, other researchers examined his findings and essentially negated the diet's effectiveness in treating children with ADHD.

Many more studies followed, but for purposes of this discussion, let's jump ahead to 2004, when David W. Schab and Nhi-Ha T. Trinh gathered fifteen double-blind placebo-controlled studies conducted to that date and performed a comprehensive, quantitative meta-analysis in an attempt to draw meaningful conclusions. This was the first meta-analysis on the subject of food colors since K.A. Kavale and S.R. Forness performed theirs in 1983, so it included many studies that had been completed in the ensuing twenty years.

The results of this work "strongly suggest an association between ingestion of AFCs and hyperactivity," their conclusion states, but the researchers called for additional studies to fill in the blanks in the global understanding of this effect.

> We recommend that future research avoid the pitfalls of many prior trials by explicitly identifying subjects' demographic characteristics; by employing specific diagnostic criteria and by identifying diagnostic subtypes and comorbidities; by identifying the concurrent use of medications; by specifying the interval between administration of AFCs and measurement of effect; by administering specific AFCs rather than mixtures; by explicitly testing the blinding of subjects; and by reporting all such information in published reports.

In a paper published in 2011, Joel T. Nigg et al. completed another meta-analysis of recent studies and determined that some children with ADHD benefit from restricting food additives including colors: "Effects of food colors were notable but susceptible to publication bias or were derived from small, nongeneralizable samples. Renewed investigation of diet and ADHD is warranted."

In 2013, after a wide range of laboratory testing on rats and mice had taken place on all nine of the FDA-approved food dyes, Kobylewski and Jacobson called for still more testing on humans to determine if the reactions found in rodents also take place in human beings. In their study, published in 2013 in the *International Journal of Occupational and Environmental Health*, they reviewed all of the studies to that date and concluded that each had provided enough warning signs about potential harm to alert the food industry that these additives could be dangerous. "The inadequacy of much of the testing and the evidence for carcinogenicity, genotoxicity, and hypersensitivity, coupled with the fact that dyes do not improve the safety or nutritional quality of foods, indicates that all of the currently used dyes should be removed from the food supply and replaced, if at all, by safer colorings," they wrote.

As recently as 2018, the American Academy of Pediatrics advised that AFCs "may be associated with exacerbation of ADHD symptoms," but even this statement of official policy is couched in indefinite language. The medical and research communities, AFC manufacturers, and the FDA remain on the fence about whether or not these additives may be detrimental to children's health.

FURTHER READINGS

Arnold, L. Eugene; Lofthouse, Nicholas; and Hurt, Elizabeth. "Artificial Food Colors and Attention Deficit/Hyperactivity Symptoms: Conclusions to Dye For." *Neurotherapeutics*, July 2012, 9(3), 599–609. Accessed Jan. 25, 2020. https://www.ncbi.nlm.nih.gov/pmc/articles/PMC3441937/#__ffn_sectitle

Batada, Ameena; and Jacobson, Michael F. "Prevalence of Artificial Food Colors in Grocery Store Products Marketed to Children." *Clinical Pediatrics*, June 6, 2016. Accessed Jan. 24, 2020. https://journals.sagepub.com/doi/abs/10.1177/0009922816651621?journalCode=cpja&

Burrows, Adam. "Palette of Our Palates: A Brief History of Food Coloring and Its Regulation." *Comprehensive Reviews in Food Science and Food Safety*, Sept. 16, 2009. Accessed Jan. 28, 2020. https://doi.org/10.1111/j.1541-4337.2009.00089.x

"Color Additives Questions and Answers for Consumers." U.S. Food and Drug Administration, Jan. 4, 2018. Accessed Jan. 24, 2020. https://www.fda.gov/food/food-additives-petitions/color-additives-questions-and-answers-consumers

Kavale, K.A.; and Forness, S.R. "Hyperactivity and Diet Treatment: A Meta-analysis of the Feingold Hypothesis." *Journal of Learning Disabilities*, 1983, 16(6), 324–330.

Kobylewski, Sarah; and Jacobson, Michael. "Food Dyes: A Rainbow of Risks." Center for Science in the Public Interest, 2010. Accessed Jan. 24, 2020. https://cspinet.org/sites/default/files/attachment/food-dyes-rainbow-of-risks.pdf

Kobylewski, Sarah; and Jacobson, Michael. "Toxicology of Food Dyes." *International Journal of Occupational and Environmental Health*, Nov. 12, 2013. Accessed Jan. 24, 2020. https://www.tandfonline.com/doi/abs/10.1179/1077352512Z.00000000034

Nigg, Joel T., et al. "Meta-Analysis of Attention-Deficit/Hyperactivity Disorder or Attention-Deficit/Hyperactivity Disorder Symptoms, Restriction Diet, and Synthetic Food Color Additives." *Journal of the American Academy of Child and Adolescent*

Psychiatry, Jan. 2012, 51(1), 86–97. Accessed Jan. 25, 2020. https://www.sciencedirect.com/science/article/abs/pii/S0890856711009531

Rohrig, Brian. "Eating With Your Eyes: The Chemistry of Food Colorings." *Chem Matters Online*, American Chemical Society, Oct. 2015. Accessed Jan. 25, 2020. https://www.acs.org/content/acs/en/education/resources/highschool/chemmatters/past-issues/2015-2016/october-2015/food-colorings.html

Schab, David W.; and Trinh, Nhi-Ha T. "Do Artificial Food Colors Promote Hyperactivity in Children with Hyperactive Syndromes? A Meta-Analysis of Double-Blind Placebo-Controlled Trials." *Journal of Developmental and Behavioral Pediatrics*, Dec. 2004, 25(6), 423–434. Accessed Jan. 24, 2020. https://journals.lww.com/jrnldbp/fulltext/2004/12000/do_artificial_food_colors_promote_hyperactivity_in.7.aspx?casa_token=NdciYj1IZrEAAAAA:yAFAg3v8KGyVSBIBHHq5buGJ2tQJyRXWrjUm7n6jB67MzbQ379I_rpV9z5-t_TQQlJ4u8_0AJeXo67_fVaGjL9Ub

Stevens, Laura, et al. "Amounts of Artificial Food Dyes and Added Sugars in Foods and Sweets Commonly Consumed By Children." *Clinical Pediatrics*, Apr. 24, 2014, 54(4), 309–321. Accessed Jan. 25, 2020. https://journals.sagepub.com/doi/abs/10.1177/0009922814530803?rfr_dat=cr_pub%3Dpubmed&url_ver=Z39.88-2003&rfr_id=ori%3Arid%3Acrossref.org&journalCode=cpja

Trasande, Leonardo, et al. "Food Additives and Child Health." *Pediatrics*, Aug. 2018, 142(2). Accessed Jan. 25, 2020. https://pediatrics.aappublications.org/content/142/2/e20181408

Artificial Sweeteners

WHAT ARE THEY?

Artificial sweeteners add sweetness to foods without adding calories or by adding a tiny fraction of the calories of sugar. Also known as nonnutritive sweeteners or sugar substitutes, the six artificial sweeteners listed by the FDA as "GRAS" include aspartame (Equal®, SugarTwin®, or NutraSweet®, packaged in blue packets), sucralose (Splenda®, packaged in yellow), and saccharin (Sweet'N Low®, SweetTwin®, or NectaSweet®, in pink packets), as well as sweeteners used primarily in packaged foods: acesulfame-potassium (Ace-K, also known as Sunett® or Sweet One®), a sweetener with a bitter aftertaste that is often combined with another artificial sweetener in food processing; neotame (Newtame®), an intense sweetener manufactured by NutraSweet, said to be fifteen times sweeter than Splenda and up to 8,000 times sweeter than sugar; and advantame, which is 20,000 times sweeter than table sugar.

Some sources also include steviol glycosides (Stevia®, green packets) as an artificial sweetener, as it occurs naturally in the leaves of the *Stevia rebaudiana* plant, but is often extracted using chemicals, particularly ethanol. The FDA lists steviol glycosides as a high-intensity sweetener (200–400 times sweeter than sugar) and considers the high-purity stevia-derived sweeteners (95 percent minimum purity) as GRAS, but stevia leaf and crude stevia extracts do not quality as GRAS and are "not permitted for use as sweeteners."

CURRENT CONSUMPTION STATISTICS AND TRENDS

The most recent scholarly study on consumption of artificial sweeteners comes from the Milken Institute School of Public Health at George Washington University, published in January 2017. The study determined that in 2012, roughly 25 percent of children in the United States and more than 41 percent of adults say that they consume foods that contain "low-calorie sweeteners," as the report calls them, including aspartame, sucralose, and saccharin. This is a significant increase over 1999, when just 8.7 percent of children and about 20 percent of adults reported choosing artificial sweeteners over sugar.

The study goes on to note that 44 percent of adults and 20 percent of children surveyed said that they ate or drank products with artificial sweeteners in them more than once a day—and 17 percent of adults said they had an artificially sweetened beverage three or more times a day. "The likelihood of consuming low-calorie sweeteners went up as adult body mass index, a measure of obesity, went up," a summary of the study said. "Nineteen percent of adults with obesity compared to 13 percent of normal weight adults used [low-calorie sweetened] products three times a day or more."

NUTRITIONAL INFORMATION

Sugar adds 16 calories per teaspoon to foods and drinks, and a 12-ounce canned soft drink that contains 39 g of sugar (usually in the form of high-fructose corn syrup, which is even more concentrated than sugar) adds about 160 calories to a meal or snack. Saccharin, sucralose, and aspartame are noncaloric and pass through the body without metabolizing, so they add no calories or carbohydrates to foods or drinks. They also gained the moniker "high-intensity sweeteners," because they are many times sweeter than sugar. Sucralose, for example, is 600 times sweeter than sugar, while stevia beats sugar's sweetness by 200–400 times. Saccharin is 300–500 times sweeter than sugar, and aspartame exceeds sugar's sweetness by 160–200 times. This means that foods and drinks require very small amounts of these sweeteners to achieve the desired sweetness—which is why a single-serving packet of sugar contains about a teaspoon (2–4 g), while a packet of Splenda contains just 12 mg of sucralose, or less than 1/100 of a teaspoon.

While artificial sweeteners have no nutritive value of their own, they are not carbohydrates, so their use can reduce the negative effects on the body of eating foods sweetened with sugar. Excessive sugar consumption causes weight gain, increases overall blood sugar levels beyond what is needed to produce energy, and can lead to obesity-related diseases including heart disease and diabetes. Artificial sweeteners do not have these effects.

HISTORY

The concept of artificial sweeteners had not risen to the scientific consciousness before 1879, when Constantine Fahlberg, a researcher at Johns Hopkins University, stumbled upon one by accident. He worked in professor Ira Remsen's laboratory and, in the midst of an experiment, spilled a chemical—a coal-tar derivative—on his hands. The very model of the absent-minded scientist, he forgot about the spill and neglected to wash his hands before dinner, and paused in mid-bite when something on his hands made the bread taste sweet. Most people might have seen this swallowing of an unknown substance as a potential threat to life and limb, but Fahlberg reacted with scientific curiosity. He returned to the lab, tasted every chemical he had used that day—again, with no regard for the very likely event that at least one may have been poisonous—and finally sipped from a beaker filled with benzoic sulfimide, which tasted sweeter than sugar. He and Remsen wrote a paper together listing them both as the creators of the new compound. In 1884, Fahlberg obtained a patent for the process that created the sweetener, which he had named saccharin, and began seeing commercial success with the new product. He essentially cut Remsen out of the business, however, leading Remsen to comment in a letter to another chemist, William Ramsey, "Fahlberg is a scoundrel. It nauseates me to hear my name mentioned in the same breath with him."

Saccharin saw some early interest, especially after Fahlberg produced the results of thousands of tests that proved it was not toxic, but the sugar beet lobby soon recognized it as a threat to Central European farmers' livelihoods. It campaigned heavily against the new substance and actually succeeded in restricting saccharin's use to pharmaceuticals, effectively ending the growth of the artificial sweeteners industry in the short term. Undaunted and well aware of the potential usefulness of his product, Fahlberg toughed out the ban until the beginning of World War I, when attitudes toward saccharin changed. In the face of sugar shortages throughout the United States and Europe, saccharin became a relatively inexpensive way to keep sweetened packaged foods on the market. Central European governments lifted the ban on its use in food, and saccharin became a massively successful product—much to Remsen's continued chagrin, though he refused an offer from pharmaceutical manufacturer Merck & Company to challenge Fahlberg's patent. Remsen's response: He "would not sully his hands with industry" (Allen & O'Shea, p. 161).

Such a popular and lucrative product could not exist as the only artificial sweetener for long. In the 1950s, sodium cyclamate—the sweetener known simply as cyclamates—arrived on the market and soon became the preferred brand for many uses, especially soft drinks. While saccharin could produce a bitter aftertaste that reminded the consumer that it was not real sugar, cyclamates had no bitterness, so it gained popularity rapidly. With increased consumption of diet drinks and snacks sweetened with the new substance, however, came an accompanying increase in bladder cancer, particularly in men. Scientists began testing cyclamates and discovered that rats in a laboratory setting developed bladder cancer when they ate large doses of the chemical. The FDA moved quickly to order all foods and drinks containing cyclamates to be removed gradually from the market, beginning in the fall of 1969. . . but the FDA allowed some use of cyclamates in diet foods made specifically for diabetics, because the organization believed that the risk of cancer was less dangerous than the risk of obesity in these patients. In 1970, it reversed this position and took cyclamates off the market altogether.

This launched a decade of more careful scrutiny of saccharin, leading to studies that seemed to point to the sweetener as another cause of bladder cancer in rodents. In 1981, saccharin was placed on the U.S. National Toxicology Program's Report on Carcinogens list, which resulted in the requirement that the makers of the artificial sweetener print a warning on any package containing saccharin, stating that this product might cause cancer. Further studies determined, however, that saccharin only causes cancer in rats, through a mechanism not found in the human body. Testing involving human subjects showed no relationship between saccharin and bladder cancer, so the sweetener came off the carcinogens list in 2000.

Aspartame entered the market in 1981, when the FDA completed its review of tests that showed that it did not cause cancer. Sucralose received its FDA approval for general use in 1998, and it was followed by acesulfame-potassium and neotame in 2002 and advantame in 2014.

THE CONTROVERSY

The scientific community has struggled to reach any kind of consensus on the health benefits versus the hazards of using artificial sweeteners in foods and drinks. Studies have produced a wide range of positive and negative results, and while claims that artificial sweeteners are carcinogens have been largely put to rest, scientists tirelessly pursue the answer to whether any or all of these sweeteners are harming the human body in other ways. Perhaps scientists believe that the idea that something that tastes so good can also improve our health is simply too good to be true, but some studies point to potentially negative effects of these sweeteners—and other studies indicate that they have no adverse effects at all.

The more salient argument is whether or not artificial sweeteners assist with weight loss. The short answer appears to be no, especially in the category of diet drinks. People who drink diet soda, for example, often make the decision to eat foods that more than make up for the calories they saved with the diet drink—for example, "I was good and ordered a diet drink, so now I can have ice cream." Some studies have suggested that the artificial sweeteners themselves cause people to gain weight, including a 2005 study conducted by the University of Texas Health Science Center at San Antonio, in which the researchers concluded that people who drank diet soda gained more weight than people who drank soda sweetened with sugar or corn syrup (DeNoon).

An even more troubling finding by S.E. Swithers and T.L. Davidson at Purdue University revealed that humans and animals use sweetness to tell them that a food is highly caloric, so that the body can gauge how much food it needs to maintain its energy. Sweet foods that contain fewer calories appear to deceive the body's energy regulation system (sugar digestion, involving insulin), so the body craves additional calories and continues to eat. This phenomenon leads to increased weight gain from eating much more of an artificially sweetened food than a person may have eaten of a food containing sugar. "A sweet taste induces an insulin response, which causes blood sugar to be stored in tissue," wrote Kirtida R. Tandel succinctly in a literature review in the *Journal of Pharmacology & Pharmacotherapeutics* in October 2011, "but because blood sugar does not increase with artificial sweeteners, there is hypoglycemia and increased food intake."

Hundreds of studies have contributed to this controversy, but many of these do not meet the standards for scientific rigor to become definitive on the subject. Studies involving mice or rats and their sweetener intake may not be relevant to human experience, as rodents digest and use sugar differently from people. Studies with a handful of subjects and few controls cannot be considered conclusive; at best, they serve as potential models for much more substantial research. Literature reviews struggle to draw conclusions because of the sheer volume of studies to review and categorize.

One recent study stands out from the rest, however. It appeared in the September 2019 issue of *JAMA Internal Medicine*, one of the peer-reviewed journals of the American Medical Association. The study uses the availability of massive amounts of data from the European Investigation into Cancer and Nutrition to review the soft drink consumption habits of 451,743 people in ten European countries, gathered from 1992 to 2000. Lengthy analysis of the data determined that people who consumed two or more soft drinks a day—sweetened with sugar or artificial sweeteners—had "higher all-cause mortality." This means that people who habitually drank soft drinks on a daily basis died during the study more frequently than people who drank less than one glass of a soft drink per month (Mullee et al.).

The study went on to break down the causes of death, based on whether the participants reported that they drank sugar-sweetened soft drinks or artificially sweetened ones. People who drank two or more diet soft drinks a day were more likely to die from a circulatory disease (stroke or heart disease), while people who drank sugary drinks died more often from digestive diseases (diabetes, kidney and liver diseases, and colorectal cancer). "Total soft drink consumption was positively associated with colorectal cancer deaths," the study said, but they could not find a correlation between soft drinks and breast or prostate cancer. "We observed no association between soft drink consumption and overall cancer mortality," the authors continued. "This result is consistent with findings in most previous studies, which found little evidence of a direct association between soft drink consumption and cancer risk."

In addition, this may be the first study to report a correlation between total soft drink consumption and a greater risk of death from Parkinson's disease. The risk is present for people who drink either sugar-sweetened or diet soft drink quantities of two per day or more.

The study stops short of suggesting that the soft drinks actually cause the diseases and only states that it found "positive associations" between the drinks and the diseases people developed. "Further studies are needed to investigate the possible adverse health effects of artificial sweeteners," it concludes.

So there continues to be no definitive answer on whether artificial sweeteners assist in weight loss or even if they trigger a glycemic response in the human body. What we do know is that the FDA considers them safe for consumption—but, like all foods, only in moderation.

FURTHER READINGS

Allen, Thomas J.; and O'Shea, Rory P. *Building Technology Transfer Within Research Universities*. Cambridge, England: Cambridge University Press, 2014, p. 159–161.

"Artificial Sweeteners and Cancer." National Cancer Institute, National Institutes of Health. Accessed Aug. 22, 2019. https://www.cancer.gov/about-cancer/causes-prevention/risk/diet/artificial-sweeteners-fact-sheet

"Consumption of Low-Calorie Sweeteners Jumps by 200 Percent in U.S. Children." George Washington University, Milken Institute School of Public Health, Jan. 10, 2017. Accessed Aug. 19, 2019. https://publichealth.gwu.edu/content/consumption-low-calorie-sweeteners-jumps-200-percent-us-children

DeNoon, Daniel J. "Drink More Diet Soda, Gain More Weight? Overweight Risk Soars 41% with Each Daily Can of Diet Soft Drink." *WebMD Medical News*, 2005.

"Healthy Lifestyle: Nutrition and Healthy Eating." Mayo Clinic. Accessed Aug. 21, 2019. https://www.mayoclinic.org/healthy-lifestyle/nutrition-and-healthy-eating/in-depth/artificial-sweeteners/art-20046936

Lyons, Richard D. "The FDA Orders a Total Cyclamate Ban." *New York Times*, Aug. 23, 1970, p. E6. Accessed Aug. 22, 2019. https://www.nytimes.com/1970/08/23/archives/the-fda-orders-a-total-cyclamate-ban-another-switch.html

Mullee, Amy, et al. "Association Between Soft Drink Consumption and Mortality in 10 European Countries." *JAMA Internal Medicine*, Sept. 3, 2019. Accessed Sept. 9, 2019. https://jamanetwork.com/journals/jamainternalmedicine/fullarticle/2749350?guestAccessKey=b99410a9-8afc-4953-b328-bbb2620dfacd&utm_source=For_The_Media&utm_medium=referral&utm_campaign=ftm_links&utm_content=tfl&utm_term=090319

Swithers, S.E.; and Davidson, T.L. "A Role for Sweet Taste: Calorie Predictive Relations in Energy Regulation by Rate." *Behavioral Neuroscience*, Feb. 2008, 122(1), 161–173. Accessed Aug. 22, 2019. https://www.ncbi.nlm.nih.gov/pubmed/18298259/

Tandel, Kirtida R. "Sugar Substitutes: Health Controversy Over Perceived Benefits." *Journal of Pharmacology & Pharmacotherapeutics*, Oct. 2011, 2(4), 236–243. Accessed Aug. 22, 2019. https://www.ncbi.nlm.nih.gov/pmc/articles/PMC3198517/

Bottled Water

WHAT IS IT?

Water in a bottle seems like the simplest product to define, but it comes from a wide range of sources and therefore requires a fairly complex set of definitions. The FDA regulates bottled water, so consumers may see a number of different classifications based on each brand's origin and additional contents.

- *Alkaline water* contains a higher level of pH than standard drinking water, which in itself has no specific benefit; but it also has negative oxidation reduction potential. This means that it acts as an antioxidant, which may make it slightly beneficial for certain health issues, including acid reflux. The potential benefits also depend on whether the water gained its alkalinity naturally (by flowing over rocks and picking up minerals) or chemically (via electrolysis in a bottling plant).
- *Artesian water* is spring water trapped under the surface by hard rock, so it cannot break through on its own. Humans gain access to it by digging a well. The water flows between rocks underground at high natural pressure, a process that acts as a natural filter. (Spring water lives underground as well, but a spring finds its way to the surface without human assistance.)
- *Distilled water* has been purified by boiling it into vapor and then condensing it back into liquid. This removes impurities, making the water safe for specific uses, like in medical equipment or appliances (e.g., use in a steam iron or CPAP machine).
- *Ionized water* has been treated with a device called an ionizer to raise its pH level, separating acidic and alkaline molecules and removing the acidic ones. This is one way to achieve the higher pH of alkaline water, which may be slightly beneficial to people with chronic acid reflux.
- *Mineral water* must be bottled at its source—natural reservoirs and mineral springs. It contains a regulated amount of dissolved minerals—more than 250 parts per million in the United States. It may contain bicarbonate, calcium, iron, magnesium, potassium, sodium, and/or zinc, and it may be processed to remove potential toxins like arsenic that it came by naturally. Sometimes carbon dioxide has been removed from it as well—and sometimes it is added to produce carbonation.
- *Purified water* (or *demineralized water*) has had impurities removed via distillation, reverse osmosis, or deionization. Many purified water suppliers use tap water to fill their bottles, purifying it to remove the unpleasant-tasting chemicals often required to treat water in municipal water systems.
- *Sparkling water (seltzer)* contains carbon dioxide that creates carbonation (bubbles). This may be plain or flavored slightly with trace amounts of fruit—more to activate the sense of smell than taste. The popular sparkling waters on the market now are zero-calorie products that contain nothing but carbonated water and scent. Some sparkling water products offer stronger fruit flavors, mixed with some kind of sweetener; most recently, "hard" seltzer spiked with alcohol has joined the water market.
- *Spring water* must come from a flowing source that begins underground and finds its own way to the planet's surface.

- *Vitamin water* (*fortified* or *enriched water*) is water to which vitamins and minerals have been added. It often contains artificial sweetener or some form of sugar (fructose, corn syrup, or cane sugar) as well as colors and flavors added by the manufacturer. Some brands have as much sugar in them as a similarly sized can of regular cola. Soft drinks masquerading as health boosters, enriched water brands contain enough nonnutritive additives to make them a poor choice for regular hydration.
- *Well water* comes from a human-made well, which in turn gets its water from an underground aquifer.

CURRENT CONSUMPTION STATISTICS AND TRENDS

In the United States in 2017, Americans consumed 42.1 gallons of bottled water per person. If we break that down by standard 16.9-ounce bottles, that averages out to a little more than 159 bottles each or a bottle every 2.2 days.

Beverage Industry magazine reported in July 2019 on a poll taken by the International Bottled Water Association earlier that year, which discovered that bottled water is the number one drink among consumers. Bottled water sales show no sign of slowing—in fact, the market continues to grow. A remarkable 72 percent of Americans said that bottled water is their preferred nonalcoholic beverage, up 9 percent from the previous year. Still water alone (as opposed to sparkling), sold in single serving bottles or as jugs for water coolers, represents a nearly $14 billion market, with the greatest share going to private label brands—store brands that are usually bottled by the big name brands, labeled for local supermarkets, and sold at lower prices than the name brands. Sparkling water adds another $3 billion to the market's total.

What is driving this juggernaut? Consumers clearly want alternatives to sweetened soft drinks like soda and juices, especially when presented with the harmful effects of high-fructose corn syrup, one of the most popular sweeteners in processed foods and drinks. At the same time, flavored waters have gained traction, including those with as much sweetener and flavoring in them as a 12-ounce can of cola.

NUTRITIONAL INFORMATION

For the most part, bottled water has no calories, and its nutritional value lies in hydration rather than in the trace amounts of calcium, sodium, or other minerals that may be found in water at the source or that may remain after filtering. Water is vital to the proper functioning of every part of the human body. It aids the bloodstream in carrying nutrients to cells, assists in digestion, prevents constipation, balances the body's electrolytes, protects organs, provides the basis for urine to flush out the bladder, and even regulates body temperature. Whether water comes from the tap or from a bottle, it provides all of these benefits—and tap water does these things just as well as bottled water.

The exception may be mineral water, which can be a source of calcium, magnesium, and potassium, things the body needs on a regular basis. Studies have shown that drinking mineral water can increase the body's levels of these minerals, which can in turn help build stronger bones, lower blood pressure, and regulate circulation and heartbeat. It may also have a relieving effect on constipation.

Some water products contain a number of additives that contribute vitamins to the body's intake. Some of these also contain flavorings, fruit juices, and sugar or sugar alcohols, which add calories. The value of the added vitamins—which are readily available in foods most people eat anyway—may be negated by the effects of the added sugar, a central component in weight gain, diabetes, and heart disease. Consumers should be careful to read the labels on these products and check the carbohydrate load to be certain that they are choosing a water product without sugar.

HISTORY

People have carried water in containers since the Roman empire and probably before that, but bottled water first became a marketable product in the United Kingdom in 1622, when the Holy Well bottling plant sold water from its mineral springs. Seeing the success of this first enterprise, other locations with mineral springs followed suit, making the water industry a new enterprise by the beginning of the 1700s. The concept came to the United States as far back as 1767, when Jackson's Spa in Boston packaged its natural spring water for sale, with the altruistic-sounding goal of sharing its supposed medicinal properties with a wider audience.

In 1783, Swiss entrepreneur Johann Jacob Schweppe found a way to carbonate water, a quality that had been restricted to natural mineral springs. American businessman Joseph Hawkins discovered the carbonation method around the same time and on his own, securing the U.S. patent for the carbonation process in 1809 and marketing bubbly water across the country. By 1856, bottled water had become a significant industry, with more than seven million bottles sold by Saratoga Springs in New York State, another spa area with natural springs believed to have healing ability. As cholera and typhoid swept through the country's cities, many people turned to bottled water as a safe way to obtain drinking water. It took until 1908 for scientists to determine that disinfection of municipal water supplies with chlorine could prevent the spread of disease. Jersey City, New Jersey, became the first city to disinfect its drinking water with chlorine, and its success led every other major water supplier to do the same, which stymied the bottled water market.

With the introduction of plastic bottling for carbonated beverages in 1973, bottled water had a chance to emerge once again. The first brand to take full advantage of this was Perrier, introduced in the United States in 1977, bringing carbonated water back to the marketing forefront. Noncarbonated (still) water came later, but its popularity grew as people began to distrust drinking fountains (perhaps during the beginning of the AIDS crisis in the early 1980s, when the method of contagion remained unknown). As bottled water became more available for less cost and municipal utilities added more chemicals that altered tap water's taste, consumers began to prefer bottled water and consider it to be better than tap. Today the industry offers hundreds of water products that, collectively, compete effectively with sweetened soft drinks.

THE CONTROVERSY

"No one should assume that just because he or she purchases water in a bottle that it is necessarily any better regulated, purer, or safer than most tap water," the Natural Resources Defense Council (NRDC) said in its report to the U.S. FDA in February 1999. The NRDC took on the issue of bottled water purity as the market for these supposedly pristine products began to ramp up, moving from barely $1 billion in sales in 1988 to more than $4 billion just ten years later. The report cited dozens of ads in magazines, in newspapers, and on television with footage of "towering mountains, pristine glaciers, and crystal-clear springs nestled in untouched forests yielding absolutely pure water." Only a fraction of the water sold in bottles, however, actually came from these unspoiled sources—in fact, much of it came out of the tap at a bottling facility. (Tap water is regulated by the Environmental Protection Agency, not the FDA, an arrangement that widens the gap between safety standards for each.)

Some bottled water even came from sources less pure than the drinking water consumers had in their own homes. "People spend from 240 to over 10,000 times more per gallon for bottled water than they typically do for tap water," the report continued, but the bottling companies deliberately misled consumers. One brand, the NRDC discovered, took its bottled water from a well in the factory's parking lot, which stood near a "hazardous waste dump, and periodically was contaminated with industrial chemicals at levels above FDA standards." The NRDC estimated that as much as 40 percent of bottled water came right out of the tap, and most of this received no additional treatment before it landed on store shelves.

How could this be? At the time, the FDA did not apply its rules for bottled water purity to water packaged and sold within the same state. Most states had their own regulations that covered these water products, but some did not. In addition, the FDA exempted carbonated water from its standards, setting "no specific contamination limits" on seltzers.

The NRDC's revealing and detailed report led to much more stringent FDA standards for bottled water, which in turn led to labeling that defined exactly where the water in the bottle had originated and what had been done to it before bottling. This is the origin of the many different classifications for bottled water we now see on store shelves. Forty states continue to regulate bottled water that is acquired and packaged within the state (and as of this writing, ten states don't bother). The new standards also strengthened the perception that bottled water in just about any form must be purer than tap water, a point of view that sent sales skyrocketing and opened the market to all kinds of new ways to purify and fortify water.

So some baselines are in place to keep bottled water relatively pure, but consumers are still left with nearly a dozen different classifications for water, some of which make startling claims about their healthfulness. This creates a difficult field to navigate, whether consumers want some kind of vitamin or mineral boost for their body's benefit or simply seek to stay hydrated.

Water labeled artesian, demineralized, purified, sparkling (plain), spring, or well water is simply water, some of which has been filtered to remove things that may affect its taste or purity. Each of these is labeled to explain its ultimate origin, while some labels provide additional information about the purification process the water has undergone since it was acquired. This still can be confusing, however, because each state regulates its own water within the state, resulting in different terminology in one state versus another. The savvy water consumer (i.e., one who has not simply installed a water filter at home, which will remove the same impurities and chemicals that water bottlers do) will read the label carefully to be sure he or she is not spending several dollars per bottle to purchase water no purer than what they already have in their home's pipes.

Water bottlers are quick to embrace ways to position their products as carriers of special health benefits. Alkaline water, for example, has attempted to play a role in bringing the benefits of antioxidants to people with high blood pressure, diabetes, high cholesterol, and acid reflux, providing an aid to cleanse the colon and achieve overall detoxification. It has been touted as a way to make the entire human body less acidic, something that sounds desirable but is actually unnecessary—the healthy human body takes care of this process itself. The body will react to too much alkalinity, though, with a condition called metabolic alkalosis, which causes nausea, vomiting, tremors, muscle twitches, confusion, and other unpleasantness.

For those who suffer from acid reflux disease, however, reduction in acidity seems like an important goal. Indeed, alkaline water may help with this condition: A laboratory study conducted in 2012 found that alkaline water with a pH of 8.8 permanently inactivated pepsin in a test tube, the substance in the body that causes acid reflux. This may be a useful discovery, said Jamie Koufman, MD, the physician who conducted this research, but she later told Microsoft News that "no science backs the claim that drinking alkaline water changes the entire pH balance of the body." This is because hydrochloric acid, one of the natural digestive chemicals in the stomach, neutralizes the pH in the water before the body can absorb it. It then disposes of any extra pH in urine, bypassing the bloodstream altogether. "You're probably better off just drinking lemon water," she concluded. The Mayo Clinic concurs, noting that more research will be required to verify any other claims made by alkaline water bottlers that their product may have a beneficial effect on cancer, heart disease, or bone loss (Zeratsky, 2019).

Many consumers have turned to sparkling waters, particularly the unsweetened but slightly flavored ones, as an alternative to sweetened soft drinks. While these seltzers offer a noncaloric option with the pleasant fizz of sodas, they do have at least one drawback: The carbonation can damage tooth enamel. A study published in 2018 in the *Korean Journal of Orthodontics* tested the effects of carbonated water on premolar teeth and found significant changes in microhardness of the teeth submerged for fifteen minutes three times a day for a week. The study concluded that carbonated water has a negative effect on etched or sealed tooth enamel.

Finally, no discussion of bottled water can be complete without addressing the effects of the bottles themselves. Plastic bottles can contain bisphenol A (BPA), a structural component in plastic, which has been in use since the 1960s. BPA has the ability to bind with estrogen in the human body, so a number of studies have explored how much BPA actually migrates from the water bottle into the consumer's body and its potential for harmful effects. Some of these studies have found trace amounts of BPA in subjects' biology, but they have not drawn conclusions about what effect this component may have on people's health. A longitudinal study currently in progress at ten universities under the auspices of the National Toxicology Program and the FDA's National Center for Toxicological Research is attempting to understand how these small amounts of BPA may affect a wide range of organs in rats. In the interim, the FDA's current advisory is that "BPA is safe at the current levels occurring in foods. Based on FDA's ongoing safety review of scientific evidence, the available information continues to support the safety of BPA for the currently approved uses in food containers and packaging."

That being said, FDA did amend its food additive regulations to eliminate the use of BPA in infant formula bottles, baby bottles, and sippy cups, because manufacturers took the step of abandoning the use of the component in their products.

FURTHER READINGS

"2019 State of the Beverage Industry: Bottled Water Remains #1." *Beverage Industry*, July 15, 2019. Accessed Aug. 23, 2019. https://www.bevindustry.com/articles/92234-2019-state-of-the-beverage-industry-bottled-water-remains-no-1

"A Brief History of Bottled Water in America." *Great Lakes Law*, Mar. 2009. Accessed Aug. 25, 2019. https://www.greatlakeslaw.org/blog/2009/03/a-brief-history-of-bottled-water-in-america.html

"Bisphenol A (BPA): Use in Food Contact Application." U.S. Food & Drug Administration. Accessed Jan. 28, 2020. https://www.fda.gov/food/food-additives-petitions/bisphenol-bpa-use-food-contact-application

DiNuzzo, Emily. "This Is What Alkaline Water Really Does to Your Body." *MSN Lifestyle, Microsoft News*, Mar. 15, 2019. Accessed Aug. 23, 2019. https://www.msn.com/en-us/health/health-news/this-is-what-alkaline-water-really-does-to-your-body/ar-BBUMWQL

Eske, Jamie. "What Are the Health Benefits of Mineral Water?" *Medical News Today*, Apr. 9, 2019. Accessed Aug. 23, 2019. https://www.medicalnewstoday.com/articles/324910.php

Goldman, Rena; and Nagelberg, Rachel. "Alkaline Water: Benefits and Risks." Healthline, May 30, 2019. Accessed Aug. 23, 2019. https://www.healthline.com/health/food-nutrition/alkaline-water-benefits-risks#benefits

Koufman, J.A.; and Johnston, N. "Potential Benefits of pH 8.8 Alkaline Drinking Water as an Adjunct in the Treatment of Reflux Disease." *Annals of Otology, Rhinology & Laryngology*, July 2012, 121(7), 431–434. Accessed Aug. 23, 2019. https://www.ncbi.nlm.nih.gov/pubmed/22844861

Olson, Erik D., with Poling, Diane; and Solomon, Gina. "Bottled Water: Pure Drink or Pure Hype?" Natural Resources Defense Council, Feb. 1999. Accessed Aug. 23, 2019. https://www.nrdc.org/sites/default/files/bottled-water-pure-drink-or-pure-hype-report.pdf

Postman, Andrew. "The Truth About Tap." Natural Resource Defense Council, Jan. 5, 2016. Accessed Aug. 23, 2019. https://www.nrdc.org/stories/truth-about-tap?gclid=CjwKCAjwnf7qBRAtEiwAseBO_DS7a3j3cnqeI-uepd8VloMC96E5n4-mV17Pw7GW9IU9b-ORzviNohoCPfsQAvD_BwE

Ryu, Hyo-kyung; Kim, Yong-do; Heo, Sung-su; and Kim, Sang-cheol. "Effect of Carbonated Water Manufactured by a Soda Carbonator on Etched or Sealed Enamel." *Korean Journal of Orthodontics*, Jan. 2018, 48(1), 48–56. Accessed Aug. 23, 2019. https://www.ncbi.nlm.nih.gov/pmc/articles/PMC5702778/

Zeratsky, Katherine. "Is Alkaline Water Better for You That Plain Water?" Mayo Clinic. Accessed Aug. 23, 2019. https://www.mayoclinic.org/healthy-lifestyle/nutrition-and-healthy-eating/expert-answers/alkaline-water/faq-20058029

Caffeine

WHAT IS IT?

Caffeine is an alkaloid compound in the class of methylxanthines, which occurs naturally in coffee, tea, cacao, and cola plants, as well as in guarana and yerba mate plants. This bitter-tasting crystal stimulates the central nervous system, increasing brain activity and making people feel more awake, energetic, and alert and even increasing their sociability and their overall sense of well-being. It also serves as a natural diuretic, increasing urination.

Pharmaceutical companies synthesize caffeine in a laboratory and add it to over-the-counter medications that would otherwise make people drowsy, including allergy medications like antihistamines. Analgesics used for migraines often contain caffeine, as its ability to constrict blood vessels in the brain can provide quick relief for these debilitating headaches. Consumers can buy concentrated caffeine tablets or capsules with brand names like No Doz® and Vivarin® to combat fatigue. Most recently, lab-synthesized caffeine has become a central ingredient in a wide range of energy drinks, from tiny bottles of 5-Hour Energy® to cans of soft drinks like Red Bull®.

In addition to its positive effects, caffeine can produce negative symptoms in people who overuse it or who have a greater sensitivity to its effects. Anxiety and "jitters" are often side effects of caffeine use. In people who have heart conditions, caffeine use can trigger palpitations, a rise in blood pressure, and other symptoms, though it has not been found to actually damage the heart.

Too much caffeine—more than 400 mg a day in a healthy person, according to the FDA—can raise blood pressure, increase heart rate, and cause sleeplessness. Frequent users can build up a tolerance to caffeine, making it necessary to take in larger amounts to achieve the desired effect. This is a sign of addiction, which can lead to significant withdrawal symptoms if caffeine use stops abruptly: severe, throbbing headaches; sleepiness, mood changes, irritability, and even vomiting.

CURRENT CONSUMPTION STATISTICS AND TRENDS

Actual usage statistics are hard to come by, but a look at sales of caffeinated beverages provides a solid picture of their use around the world.

- The *Journal of the American Dietetic Association* published a 2005 paper that stated that 90 percent of the world's population uses caffeine regularly. Most of these people take in about 200 mg per day—the approximate equivalent of two cups of coffee.
- The International Coffee Organization reports that from July 1, 2018, to June 30, 2019, worldwide coffee bean exports totaled 168.77 million bags, with a bag weighing 132.276 pounds (60 kg). That's a total of 22.3 billion pounds of coffee beans. This represents an 8 percent increase over the previous year, indicating that coffee consumption is rising.
- The market for tea in the United States continues to expand by 6.9 percent annually, with a predicted $214.7 million in 2019. These figures are limited to black and green tea, both of which are usually caffeinated; they do not include herbal, instant, iced, or ready-to-drink teas.
- Coca-Cola reports that worldwide consumers drink more than 1.9 billion cans and bottles of their products every day. While not all of these products are caffeinated—Coke owns a number of caffeine-free beverages and bottled water brands—Coca-Cola's original cola brand continues to be the number one selling soft drink in the United States.
- The popularity of energy drinks continues to rise, with 6.8 billion cans of Red Bull sold worldwide in 2018. The National Center for Complementary and Integrative Health reports that energy drinks are "the most popular dietary supplement consumed by American teens and young adults," second only to multivitamins. Men between the ages of eighteen and thirty-four are the largest audience for these drinks, with adolescents between twelve and seventeen years the next biggest group of consumers.

NUTRITIONAL INFORMATION

Generally, an 8-ounce cup of coffee contains somewhere between 80 and 100 mg of caffeine. A cup of black or green tea may contain 30–50 mg, while a 12-ounce can of a caffeinated soft drink usually provides 30–40 mg.

Energy drinks contain a great deal more caffeine than a typical cup of coffee. A 16-ounce can of Monster Energy or Rockstar energy drink, for example, contains 160 mg of caffeine, while a 24-ounce can of Rockstar Punched provides 360 mg of caffeine.

Beyond its value as a stimulant, caffeine does not provide any nutritional content.

HISTORY

The discovery of a stimulant in certain plants predates recorded history, so there's no way to know who first determined that coffee beans, tea leaves, or cacao beans could be used as a pick-me-up. Anthropologists make an educated guess that these plants may have come to the attention of human beings as far back as 70,000 BC, with prehistoric people chewing the seeds and roots to enjoy their stimulating properties.

Grinding beans may have become an easier way to access the benefits, but the process of infusing the plant material with boiling water is a far more recent phenomenon. We know that the Olmec civilization in what is now southern Mexico grew cacao and introduced the Mayan civilization to the beans somewhere around 300 BC. The Mayans, in turn, ground the beans and made them into a drink consumed only by those of the elite class. They shared it with the Aztecs, who decided it needed something more . . . so they added sugar and milk, and created the basis for what became the most popular confection in the world. (There's much more about the evolution of chocolate later in this book.)

There is no written record of the first time someone ground coffee beans and infused them with boiling water, but we do know that the use of coffee and tea plants for their ability to sharpen thinking and supply energy does seem to have increased dramatically in the fifteenth and sixteenth centuries, right about when explorers from the European nations set out to find routes to exotic locales in South America, Africa, and the Far East. By the 1600s, as ships returned to Europe fairly regularly from these regions, drinks featuring caffeine had begun to grow in popularity among the upper classes. For the most part, however, coffee and tea were seen as part of the apothecary, not a staple at breakfast or the finish of a nice meal. Robert Burton's staggeringly extensive medical text, *The Anatomy of Melancholy*, first published in 1621, discusses coffee as a medicine. He notes its usefulness in producing an antidote to melancholy, its worth as a stimulant, and its positive effect on digestion. This usage persisted throughout the fifteenth century, with physicians of the time crediting coffee as a cure for everything from coughs and colds to the bubonic plague.

Tea, meanwhile, may have originated in China around 3000 BC. The legend goes that when Shennong, the emperor at the time, accidentally dropped some leaves into boiling water, he noted that they produced a pleasing aroma. He sampled the resulting beverage and not only enjoyed the flavor, but he recognized the burst of energy he felt shortly thereafter as coming from the tea. Civilizations in other parts of the world discovered tea in their own time: archaeologists have found it in the relics of Native American tribes dating back thousands of years, so it's conceivable that tea emerged in the western hemisphere concurrently with its use in Asia.

Tea also served as a medicinal drink—in fact, the only way it was permitted into England during the Cromwell Protectorate in the mid-1600s was as a curative for various ailments. By this time, Chinese physicians had used tea leaves sanitized in boiling water as a tonic since AD 350, further confirming its usefulness. Once the protectorate dissolved and imports from China became more regular, tea grew to become the drink of choice in the United Kingdom, putting it on a parallel path with coffee for the most desired caffeinated drink.

One testament to coffee's quickly growing popularity in Europe is the "Coffee Cantata," a composition by Johann Sebastian Bach, written in 1734 to lyrics supplied by poet Picander. The song celebrates Zimmerman's Coffee House in Germany, where Bach and his students often performed:

> Ah! How sweet the coffee's taste is,
> Sweeter than a thousand kisses,
> Milder than sweet muscatel.
> Coffee, coffee, I must have it,
> And if someone wants to treat me,
> Ah, my cup with coffee fill!

Something so beneficial to concentration and productivity could only gain momentum, so by the nineteenth century, coffee and tea held places in every corner of society. Still, the specific element that gave these drinks their energy-boosting ability had not yet been discovered.

In 1819, a German chemist named Friedlieb Ferdinand Runge isolated the compound in coffee that provided the energy and medicinal value and named it *kaffebase*—translating to "coffee base." Word did not travel around the world the way it does today, of course, so when three scientists in France isolated the chemical independently in 1821, they felt they could lay claim to the discovery. Pierre Jean Robiquet, Pierre-Joseph Pelletier, and Joseph Bienaimé Caventou did receive their places in history, as they apparently arrived at their conclusions without any knowledge of Runge's work. Robiquet managed to make the first presentation of the discovery at the Pharmacy Society meeting later that year, so he received the accolades; meanwhile, Pelletier published an article in which he named the compound caffeine, sealing his own spot in the annals of history.

Germany claimed one more scientific victory in the development of caffeine as a marketable commodity: Chemist Hermann Emil Fischer became the first to synthesize the compound in a laboratory, making it possible to create caffeine without the costly process of harvesting plants that only grow in exotic locations. He received the Nobel Prize in 1902 for his work in chemical reactions and processes for synthesizing chemicals. (In a remarkable feat of symmetry, he is also the discoverer of barbiturates—sedatives used to combat insomnia.)

With a process for synthesizing caffeine at the ready, mass production and marketing of all manner of caffeinated beverages could begin. By the twentieth century, "the cultural life of caffeine, as transmitted through the consumption of coffee and tea, had become so interwoven with the social habits and artistic pursuits of the Western world that the coffee berry had become the biggest cash crop on earth, and tea had become the world's most popular drink," wrote Bennett A. Weinberg and Bonnie K. Bealer in their book *The World of Caffeine: The Science and Culture of the World's Most Popular Drug.*

THE CONTROVERSY

People use caffeine because of its pleasant effects, so it may come as no surprise that the drug has been credited with all kinds of benefits to body and mind. In recent years, scientists have begun to test claims about caffeine's potential medicinal uses. An article on the caffeine-centered website CaffeineInformer.com touts the "Top 25+ Caffeine Health Benefits," with links to studies—some credible, some less so—that suggest that caffeine helps grow hair on men's heads, relieves pain, prevents skin cancer, protects against cataracts, and reverses Alzheimer's disease.

Many of these studies look at data rather than performing research on actual patients. While examining lifestyle and habits of patients can be a perfectly valid way to determine a correlation between variables, more research would be required to make the leap from correlation to causation. An examination of caffeine consumption in patients who have a specific genetic marker for Parkinson's disease, for example, appears to show that patients who consume caffeine had a significantly lower risk of actually developing the disease than people who do not use caffeine. "Whether there is an actual biological interaction between caffeine mediated downstream pathways needs to be further investigated in both *in vitro* studies and in animal models," the study's authors noted (Prakash, 2015).

The claim that caffeine will grow hair comes from a study involving scalp biopsies from fourteen men who were experiencing male pattern baldness. The biopsies were tested in a laboratory, first with testosterone, resulting in "significant growth suppression," and then with tiny amounts of caffeine. "Caffeine alone led to a significant stimulation of hair follicle growth," the report noted (Fischer, 2007). Since then, hair products containing caffeine have come to market, and a 2017 study conducted in India and Germany followed 210 men for six months to see if caffeine could be as effective as minoxidil, the approved treatment for hair loss. Caffeine applied topically to the hair follicles did indeed seem nearly as effective. Just drinking beverages with caffeine does not deliver enough of the drug to grow hair, however; scientists note that about 6,000 mg of caffeine would have to be ingested daily, which is far more than anyone can take in safely.

Stories have circulated over the last several years about caffeine's role in preventing liver cancer. The most recent credible studies (i.e., with no apparent involvement of the coffee industry) suggest that coffee—not caffeine—may reduce the risk of liver cancer and other liver diseases by as much as 40 percent (Tamura, 2018). In addition, a 2010 study at the University of Maryland determined that caffeine eye drops given to rats with cataracts prevented progression of their cataracts, while rats that received a placebo eye drop had more severe cataracts (Shambhu, 2010). These results have been replicated in further studies involving humans, including one in 2019. Drinking beverages with caffeine appears to help as well, as a 2016 study noted.

Caffeine may have many pharmaceutical uses, but its psychoactive effect on the body classifies it as a drug, and drug abuse leads to negative effects. Unregulated and legal in every country, caffeine has taken a place as the most widely used drug in the world, even more so than alcohol or nicotine. Addiction is a distinct possibility, as is building up a tolerance to caffeine's stimulating effect, requiring more and more intake to achieve the desired "high."

The FDA recommends that caffeine users limit their consumption to 400 mg a day (or less). This amounts to four or five cups of coffee or up to ten 12-ounce cans of a caffeinated soft drink or as many as thirteen cups of tea. Energy drinks meet the 400-mg limit with less than three 16-ounce cans per day or with just one 24-ounce can of an "amped" energy drink. A standard bottle of an energy shot drink (such as 5-Hour Energy) delivers about 215 mg or just over half the RDA of caffeine.

Users who stay under the FDA's recommended intake may see more benefits than drawbacks to caffeine use. Caffeine used responsibly can help with weight loss, sharpen thinking, increase alertness, and improve mood. Most users have nothing to fear from a couple of cups of coffee a day unless they are particularly sensitive to caffeine's effect. People who experience tremors in their hands, increased anxiety, or palpitations from caffeine consumption may be more comfortable without the additional stimulation. None of these symptoms are permanent, so they will subside once the caffeine has run its course.

As with all drugs, however, caffeine can become destructive when abused. Teens and young adults who drink highly caffeinated energy drinks on a habitual basis are likely to take more risks, experience more depression, and see increases in blood pressure. (Many of these drinks are also high in sugar, which increases the risk of heart disease and type 2 diabetes.) The Center for Behavioral Health Statistics and Quality released a report in 2013 on the increase in the number of emergency room visits that resulted from overuse of energy drinks: Emergency visits doubled from 2007 to 2011, to more than 20,000 visits, with symptoms including insomnia, nervousness and anxiety, headache, seizures, and pounding heartbeat. "This report validates claims that energy drinks can be dangerous when used alone or in combination with other drugs or alcohol," author Margaret E. Mattson, PhD, concluded.

The *Journal of Caffeine Research* published an extensive literature review in 2013 on caffeine use disorder (also known as caffeine dependence syndrome), a clinical condition recognized by the World Health Organization. The paper describes the disorder as

> a cluster of behavioral, cognitive, and physiological phenomena that develop after repeated substance use and which typically include a strong desire to take the drug, difficulties in controlling use, persisting in use despite harmful consequences, a higher priority given to drug use than to other activities and obligations, increased tolerance, and sometimes a physical withdrawal state.
>
> (Meredith et al., 2013)

People with this disorder have become physically dependent on the drug and cannot reduce their usage, even when they know their caffeine consumption causes health issues. Moderate caffeine use can produce withdrawal symptoms including headache, fatigue, lowered mood, and trouble focusing on a task, and these send users running back to the coffeemaker for another cup. When a heavy caffeine user experiences withdrawal, it can come with throbbing migraine headaches, nausea and vomiting, depression, and more—and the desire to return to the elevated mood and functionality that caffeine brings may become permanent, even after the physical dependence has been overcome.

How big a problem is caffeine dependence? Studies have not produced a clear response to this question to date, with some suggesting that only about 6 percent of all caffeine users may have this disorder and another noting that it may be as high as 30 percent. There are enough cases to fill meetings of the 12-step Caffeine Addicts Anonymous program across the country, although the participants in these meetings self-select to attend, so their definitions of caffeine dependence may vary widely.

FURTHER READINGS

"Caffeine: Facts, Usage, and Side Effects." *Caffeine Informer*. Accessed Aug. 26, 2019. https://www.caffeineinformer.com/caffeine-trimethylxanthine

"The Company Behind the Can." Red Bull. Accessed Aug. 26, 2019. https://energydrink-us.redbull.com/en/company

"Consumption of Caffeinated Energy Drinks Rises in the United States." *Science Daily*, Apr. 29, 2019. Accessed Aug. 27, 2019. https://www.sciencedaily.com/releases/2019/04/190429125416.htm

"Energy Drinks." National Center for Complementary and Integrative Health. Accessed Aug. 26, 2019. https://nccih.nih.gov/health/energy-drinks

Fray, C.D.; Johnson, R.K.; and Wang, M.Q. "Food Sources and Intakes of Caffeine in the Diets of Persons in the United States." *Journal of the American Dietetic Association*, Jan. 2005, 105(1), 110–113. Accessed Aug. 27, 2019. https://www.ncbi.nlm.nih.gov/pubmed/15635355/

International Coffee Organization. Accessed Aug. 26, 2019. http://www.ico.org
Kumar, Prakash M., et al. "Differential Effect of Caffeine Intake in Subjects with Genetic Susceptibility to Parkinson's Disease." *Scientific Reports*, Nov. 2, 2015, 5. Accessed Aug. 27, 2019. https://www.nature.com/articles/srep15492
Mattson, Margaret E. "Update on Emergency Department Visits Involving Energy Drinks: A Continuing Public Health Concern." The CBHSQ Report, Substance Abuse and Mental Health Services Administration, Jan. 10, 2013. Accessed Aug. 27, 2019. https://www.ncbi.nlm.nih.gov/books/NBK384664/
Meredith, Steven E., et al. "Caffeine Use Disorder: A Comprehensive Review and Research Agenda." *Journal of Caffeine Research*, Sept. 2013, 3(3), 114–130. Accessed Aug. 27, 2019. https://www.ncbi.nlm.nih.gov/pmc/articles/PMC3777290/
"Spilling the Beans: How Much Caffeine Is Too Much?" U.S. Food & Drug Administration, Dec. 12, 2018. Accessed Aug. 26, 2019. https://www.fda.gov/consumers/consumer-updates/spilling-beans-how-much-caffeine-too-much
Tamura, T., et al. "Coffee, Green Tea, and Caffeine Intake and Liver Cancer Risk: A Prospective Cohort Study." Nutrition and Cancer, 2018 Nov-Dec: 70(8), 1210–1216. Accessed 27 Aug 2019. https://www.ncbi.nlm.nih.gov/pubmed/30457014
Varma, Shambhu D., et al. "Effectiveness of Topical Caffeine in Cataract Prevention: Studies with Galactose Cataract." *Molecular Vision*, Dec. 2, 2010, 16, 2626–2633. Accessed Aug. 27, 2019. http://www.molvis.org/molvis/v16/a281/
Weinberg, Bennett Alan; and Bealer, Bonnie K. *The World of Caffeine: The Science and Culture of the World's Most Popular Drug*. New York: Routledge, 2001.

Carbonated Beverages

WHAT ARE THEY?

Carbonated beverages contain dissolved carbon dioxide added to liquid under high pressure. When the pressure is released, the carbon dioxide produces bubbles (effervescence). Fizzy soft drinks (soda pop), sparkling water, some mineral waters, sparkling wine, and others are all carbonated beverages. Some of these (mineral water in particular) come by their bubbles naturally in underground springs, but most obtain their carbon dioxide through an industrial process.

CURRENT CONSUMPTION STATISTICS AND TRENDS

Many carbonated beverages contain sugar in some form, whether it is high-fructose corn syrup, cane sugar, fructose, sucrose, or one of many other kinds of highly caloric sweetener. With the availability of information about the link between sugary drinks and obesity, diabetes, and heart disease, consumption of these beverages has declined steadily since 2003, according to the ongoing

National Health and Nutrition Examination Survey. That being said, a survey published in 2017 determined that 50 percent of adults and 60.7 percent of children in the United States drank a sugary beverage daily. While these figures were down from previous years (79.7 percent of children and 61.5 percent of adults in 2003), they still represent a multibillion-dollar industry.

Instead, many consumers have chosen sparkling water as their go-to beverage, a carbonated product that contains nothing but water and carbon dioxide. Some sparkling water products also contain noncaloric flavors, which manifest mostly as scents to provide a mild sense of flavor without adding sugar. Nielsen Retail Measurement Services, the tracker of barcode scans at the register for many industries, notes that from 2014 to 2018, the sparkling water category grew 54 percent. According to Nielsen, from August 1, 2017, through July 28, 2018, sales of sparkling water hit $2.2 billion, and canned carbonated water—including the many flavored varieties—grew 43 percent over the previous year. In one week alone in the summer of 2018, Nielsen clocked sales of more than $21 million for canned sparkling water.

NUTRITIONAL INFORMATION

Carbonated water is just water, so it has no nutritional content in and of itself. As a key to hydration, it provides all of the hydration value of plain (still) water, with the added refreshment of fizz.

Carbonated soft drinks may contain high levels of sugar and sodium, both of which can have a detrimental impact on health. Drinks that are high in sugar and salt contribute to heart disease, type 2 diabetes, stroke, and other illnesses brought on by obesity.

HISTORY

Joseph Priestly, an English philosopher and chemist, earned his place in history with his discovery of oxygen and carbon monoxide, but his exploration of the "airs" we breathe eventually led him to infuse water with carbon dioxide in 1767. The resulting bubbly water did not become the focus of his work, but it held more interest for Torbern Bergman, a Swedish chemist who discovered carbonation independently in 1771 and apparently without knowledge of Priestly's discovery. He used sulfuric acid in chalk to create a process for carbonation, but he also did not see a lot of practical application for this technique and soon moved on to other experiments.

In 1783, J.J. Schweppe invented a way to produce carbonated water on a large scale. His method quickly drew the attention of other entrepreneurs, including Augustine Thwaites, an Irishman who was the first to call the beverage "soda water." The novel beverage's popularity grew as various businesses sprang up to offer it, each adding a wide range of flavors to attract customers away from competitors and into their own establishments.

It took American inventor John Matthews to build a machine in 1832 that could infuse plain water with carbon dioxide and then sell that machine to businesses, to turn carbonated beverages into a mass-market enterprise. By this time, flavored fizzy drinks had come to America with fruit flavors as well as sarsaparilla, birch bark, and dandelion, but the availability of Matthews' machine turned every pharmacy store into a soda fountain. Soon consumers wanted to be able to enjoy their soda pop at home, so inventors began working to find a way to keep the pressurized drinks in bottles without their going flat. This feat required many incremental patents until 1892, when William Painter of Baltimore created what he named the Crown Cork Bottle Seal, the first bottle top that preserved the fizz. Seven years later, Libby Glass Company patented a bottle that could be mass produced, the brainchild of staff inventor Michael Owens. Carbonated beverages soon arrived on store shelves, and in the 1920s, six-pack design and vending machines became the breakthrough inventions that brought soft drinks into every household, automobile, and workplace in the country.

THE CONTROVERSY

Carbonation has been blamed for a wide range of health issues in the popular press, from acid reflux to bone density loss and tooth enamel decay. Some of these claims result from a misreading of clinical studies in which reporters generalized the results of tests to include all carbonated beverages, instead of the soft drinks that actually contribute to the health issue.

For example, a 2006 study published in the *American Journal of Clinical Nutrition* did its best to clarify its own results with the title, "Colas, but Not Other Carbonated Beverages, Are Associated with Low Bone Mineral Density in Older Women." This study, conducted as part of the Framingham Osteoporosis Study at Tufts University, discovered that cola drinks actively reduced bone density in the hips of postmenopausal women, while other carbonated beverages did not. (See Phosphorus-Containing Food Additives for more on this.)

The claim that carbonated beverages may contribute to gastroesophageal reflux disease (GERD, also known as acid reflux) has also been proved false. Carbonation may create pressure in the stomach that relaxes the lower sphincter of the esophagus, which may temporarily irritate the esophagus if acid reflux is already present. A study conducted at the University of Arizona in 2010 and published in the peer-reviewed *Alimentary Pharmacology and Therapeutics*, however, tested and discredited the rumor that carbonation actively causes GERD. The researchers discovered that carbonation creates "a very short decline in intra-oesophageal pH," but "there is no evidence that carbonated beverages directly cause oesophageal damage. . . . Furthermore, there is no evidence that these popular drinks lead to GERD complications or oesophageal cancer."

News that carbonated beverages cause kidney stones received the same kind of media distortion, even though the study that determined this actually focused on cola. The phosphoric acid in cola beverages increases the risk of chronic kidney disease, a study of data from 465 patients in North Carolina determined. The study, published in the journal *Epidemiology*, concluded that people who drank two or more colas per day (we can assume that this refers to the standard 12-ounce cans) had an increased risk of chronic kidney disease, whether they drank full-strength sugared cola or artificially sweetened varieties. The presence of carbonation was not a factor in the higher risk. "Noncola carbonated beverages were not associated with chronic kidney disease," the study concluded.

The one area in which carbonation has a mildly damaging effect is in tooth enamel. Carbonation produces carbonic acid, which lowers a beverage's pH. This can contribute to the erosion of the coating on the outside of teeth. Beverages with a pH below 4.0—more than 93 percent of carbonated beverages, according to a study published in the *Journal of the American Dental Association* in 2016—are more corrosive than those with a pH above 4. For the most part, sparkling waters—the ones without sugar or other additives—had a pH of above 4.0, earning them a ranking of "minimally corrosive." The American Dental Association concurs with this, sharing the results of a study on teeth that were donated for research, in which they were tested to see if sparkling water was more corrosive than regular still water. "The two forms of water were about the same in their effects on tooth enamel," the ADA summarized. "This finding suggests that even though sparkling water is slightly more acidic than ordinary water, it's all just water to your teeth." The ADA still recommends plenty of regular, fluoridated water for tooth health, but sparkling water is a good alternative to sugary drinks.

In summary, the bubbles are not the problem; it's the sugar and sodium in most carbonated drinks and the acidic nature of cola that have the most destructive effects on the human body.

FURTHER READINGS

Bellis, Mary. "Introduction to Pop: The History of Soft Drinks." ThoughtCo., June 26, 2019. Accessed Aug. 28, 2019. https://www.thoughtco.com/introduction-to-pop-the-history-of-soft-drinks-1991778

"Get the Facts: Sugar-Sweetened Beverages and Consumption." Centers for Disease Control and Prevention. Accessed Aug. 28, 2019. https://www.cdc.gov/nutrition/data-statistics/sugar-sweetened-beverages-intake.html

"Invention of Carbonation and History of Carbonated Water." History of Soft Drinks. Accessed Aug. 28, 2019. http://www.historyofsoftdrinks.com/soft-drink-history/history-of-carbonated-water/

"Is Sparkling Water Bad for My Teeth?" Mouth Healthy, American Dental Association. Accessed Aug. 28, 2019. https://www.mouthhealthy.org/en/nutrition/food-tips/the-truth-about-sparkling-water-and-your-teeth?_ga=2.209146898.1056501.1567015881-730615661.1567015881

Johnson, T., et al. "Systematic Review: The Effects of Carbonated Beverages of Gastro-oesophageal Reflux Disease." *Alimentary Pharmacology and Therapeutics*, Feb. 9, 2010.

Accessed Aug. 28, 2019. https://onlinelibrary.wiley.com/doi/full/10.1111/j.1365-2036.2010.04232.x

Lambert, C.P., et al. "Fluid Replacement After Dehydration: Influence of Beverage Carbonation and Carbohydrate Content." *International Journal of Sports Medicine*, 1992, 13(4), 285–292. Accessed Aug. 28, 2019. https://www.thieme-connect.com/products/ejournals/abstract/10.1055/s-2007-1021268

"NoSignsofFizzingOut:America'sLoveofSparklingWaterRemainsStrongThroughAugust." Nielsen, Aug. 24, 2018. Accessed Aug. 28, 2019. https://www.nielsen.com/us/en/insights/article/2018/no-signs-of-fizzing-out-americas-love-of-sparkling-water-remains-strong/

Reddy, Avanija, et al. "The pH of Beverages in the United States." *Journal of the American Dental Association*, Apr. 2016, 147(4), 255–263. Accessed Aug. 28, 2019. https://jada.ada.org/article/S0002-8177%2815%2901050-8/abstract?_ga=2.77880468.1056501.1567015881-730615661.1567015881

Saldana, Tina M., et al. "Carbonated Beverages and Chronic Kidney Disease." *Epidemiology*, July 2007, 18(4), 501–506. Accessed Aug. 28, 2019. https://www.ncbi.nlm.nih.gov/pmc/articles/PMC3433753/

Specktor, Brandon. "Is Sparkling Water as Healthy as Regular Water?" *LiveScience*, Apr. 19, 2018. Accessed Aug. 28, 2019. https://www.livescience.com/62351-does-sparkling-water-hydrate-you.html

Tucker, Katherine, et al. "Colas, But Not Other Carbonated Beverages, Are Associated with Low Bone Density in Older Women: The Framingham Osteoporosis Study." *The American Journal of Clinical Nutrition*, Oct. 2006, 84(4), 936–942. Accessed Aug. 28, 2019. https://academic.oup.com/ajcn/article/84/4/936/4632980

Carrageenan

WHAT IS IT?

Carrageenan is a substance derived from red seaweed—also known as Irish moss—that is used to thicken and preserve a number of foods. You may see it listed in the ingredients of yogurt products, processed meats, milk made from nuts or soy, ice cream, whipped toppings, baby formula, chocolate milk, fancy coffee beverages, coffee creamer, and dairy products like cottage cheese and sour cream.

The market for carrageenan extends to the cosmetics and pharmaceutical industry, but dairy products and meats tend to see the largest share of usage. In particular, carrageenan keeps whey from separating out of cottage cheese and ice cream, a problem that comes from additives used in these products for other purposes. In the delicatessen (and also in pet foods), carrageenan helps retain soluble protein in hams and processed meats, binding the proteins and keeping these products intact.

CURRENT CONSUMPTION STATISTICS AND TRENDS

The entire world uses carrageenan as a product in food production, to the tune of U.S. $864.3 million in 2019. This momentum drove Mordor Intelligence to forecast that the global market will reach U.S. $1.45 billion by 2024. The world's demand for processed foods with organic ingredients drives the upward thrust of this market, with carrageenan's overall versatility and effectiveness making it the most popular thickener, gelling agent, and stabilizer for dairy products and meats, as well as a wide range of other foods. As countries in the Asia Pacific region ratchet up their own demand for prepackaged foods in recent years, the carrageenan market can expect to continue to expand.

NUTRITIONAL INFORMATION

Carrageenan does not add calories to food; nor does it add fat, sodium, cholesterol, or any other nutrient. Its contribution comes in supporting thick, creamy texture, stabilizing dairy products, and making low-fat and low-sugar foods feel as good in our mouths as their full-fat analogs. It also adds fiber, allowing foods that would otherwise have no fiber content to gain this healthful benefit.

HISTORY

To obtain carrageenan, food scientists follow a simple process that has been in use since the fifteenth century: They boil the seaweed, filter the carrageenan out of the broth, dry it, and mill it until they have a powder that can be mixed into many different foods. This is the process used by Irish cooks as far back as the 1400s, when they employed it to thicken soups and puddings, according to FoodScienceMatters.com.

Carrageenan's use dates back even farther than that, however. Archaeologists have discovered evidence among ancient relics in Chile that preserving seaweed and its by-products took place thousands of years before the modern era. The Chinese farmed seaweed in 2700 BC, and they began using red algae as a medicine around 600 BC. Antiquated Irish records note the use of the seaweed by-product as a thickener by 400 BC, and in the 1400s, seaweed became a staple in Korean cooking. Its use as a commercial thickener began in the mid-1800s in the United States, when an Irishman named Daniel Ward recognized the red seaweed in the waters off the coast of Massachusetts. He established his family's home in Scituate, Massachusetts, and began harvesting the plant using the old family method. Soon his enterprise grew to include many other Irish immigrants, who worked together to harvest the steady supply of "Irish moss" and boil it down for the valued powder.

Nearly 100 years passed before carrageenan became the dominant thickener in food processing—and like many other products, it came to the fore during a world war. With the United States at war with Japan, the supply of agar, a thickener derived from a red algae that grows in the waters off Japan's shores, became limited enough to curtail production of a number of foods. The Scituate enterprise stood ready, however, to do its patriotic duty and replace the need for agar with the more versatile carrageenan. By the time the war ended, the food industry had embraced carrageenan as its primary thickener, and U.S. suppliers met the demand by reaching out to the warm waters of the South Pacific Ocean for mass cultivation of the appropriate seaweed. This brought new industry to countries in the Indian Ocean and around the Pacific Rim, creating jobs for many people who were struggling to survive after the war. Today carrageenan production is a major industry in a number of developing countries, involving up to 100,000 families on five continents in the global enterprise.

THE CONTROVERSY

Despite carrageenan's benefits to food appearance and texture, its natural origins, and the gentle process with which its harvesters extract it from seaweed, carrageenan has become the subject of considerable controversy since 1973. The story of carrageenan's rocky relationship with scientists, bloggers, health-food enthusiasts, and Internet rumormongers begins with that most dreaded phenomenon of modern times: questionable science.

As early as 1973, the results of studies began to emerge that suggested that certain forms of carrageenan caused lesions in the colon and liver toxicity in mice and rats. In 1976, Vinegar et al. devised a process for creating inflammation in rats with carrageenan, a necessary step before using the rats to test all manner of drugs and other substances that reduce or otherwise affect swelling (edema) and inflammation. The fact that carrageenan could be used in this manner represented a warning signal for some scientists, who began studying this common food additive with more directed scrutiny. It's important to note that the process of causing inflammation in rats calls for injection of carrageenan, not consumption, so the effect on the rat's body is different from what happens in a human's digestive tract. In addition, the form of carrageenan used in this manner is "degraded" carrageenan, later renamed poligeenan by the United States Adopted Names Council. Poligeenan is a polymer used in laboratories and in clinical diagnostics—for example, to suspend barium sulfate in a slurry for X-rays of the digestive tract. It is never used in food.

It may be no surprise that such a substance caused internal lesions in rodents, but this has nothing at all to do with food-grade carrageenan. In fact, by 1974 scientists had begun testing the carrageenan used in food in parallel studies on mice, including one in which they fed mice skim milk that contained carrageenan for six months. The mice remained healthy and cancer-free, as did rats and hamsters that received varying dose levels of the carrageenan food additive in their daily diet throughout their lifespan. "From the results of this experiment, carrageenan demonstrated no carcinogenic effects in either species," the latter report concluded (Rustia, p. 1).

Studies using degraded carrageenan continued, however, and in 2001, Joanne K. Tobacman at the University of Iowa led several studies in which she concluded that carrageenan caused breast, colon, and gastrointestinal cancer. She wrote in an article in *Environmental Health Perspectives* in 2001:

> Although the International Agency for Research on Cancer in 1982 identified sufficient evidence for the carcinogenicity of degraded carrageenan in animals to regard it as posing a carcinogenic risk to humans, carrageenan is still used widely as a thickener, stabilizer, and texturizer in a variety of processed foods prevalent in the Western diet.

Degraded carrageenan had officially been renamed poligeenan in 1988 to make the distinction between it and the carrageenan used in food, but Tobacman continued to generalize the two different substances as if they were the same. The argument for this, some scientists have said, is that food-grade carrageenan degrades in the gastrointestinal system to become poligeenan. "Because of the acknowledged carcinogenic properties of degraded carrageenan in animal models and the cancer-promoting effects of undegraded carrageenan in experimental models, the widespread use of carrageenan in the Western diet should be reconsidered," Tobacman wrote.

In 2008, Tobacman petitioned the FDA to remove carrageenan from its GRAS status. The FDA reviewed the case and all of the science on both sides of the issue and finally issued a letter in 2012, reiterating the additive's qualifications for GRAS status. Carrageenan has maintained that status since then, even though Tobacman continues to research the additive and published studies as recently as June 2019 that link the additive with cancer in rodents.

One of the organizations siding with Tobacman is the Cornucopia Institute, which "provides needed information to family farmers, consumers and other stakeholders in the good food movement and to the media," according to its website. Cornucopia published a report in 2013 titled, "Carrageenan: How a 'Natural' Food Additive Is Making Us Sick," in which it summarizes the studies up to that point and expresses concern that "the acid environment of the stomach may 'degrade' food-grade carrageenan once it enters the digestive system, thus exposing the intestines to this potent and widely recognized carcinogen." It continues, "The unique chemical structure of carrageenan triggers an innate immune response in the body, which recognizes it as a dangerous invader. This immune response leads to inflammation."

Contrast this point of view with the results of a 2016 study published in *Food and Toxicology* and led by James M. McKim Jr., another expert in carrageenan research, who spent two years attempting to replicate Tobacman's findings in a study sponsored by the International Food Additive Council (IFAC). The study's conclusion: Carrageenan "has no impact on the human body when consumed in food," said Robert Rankin, IFAC's executive director, in a news release about the study. "Carrageenan producers have taken very seriously claims that the ingredient is unsafe, thoroughly investigated the research supporting those claims and found them to be baseless."

"For every seemingly irrefutable point, there seems to be an equally valid counterpoint," wrote "Nutrition Diva" Monica Reinagel, MS, LD/N, CNS, in a column in *Scientific American* about the controversy. "Individuals continue to report dramatic improvement of long-standing digestive issues when they eliminate carrageenan from their diets. Activists continue to call for a ban. The food industry continues to defend its use, citing the conclusions of scientists and government agencies. What's a consumer to do?"

So the controversy continues. On one side, groups like the Cornucopia Institute brandish Tobacman's research and insist that carrageenan is a cancer-causing agent. On the other side, IFAC and others grip McKim's research and call Tobacman's work "bad science." The one thing we know for certain is that some people who have irritable bowel syndrome, ulcerative colitis, Crohn's disease, or other gastrointestinal issues find foods that contain carrageenan to be irritating to their condition. If you have one of these illnesses, consider reducing your intake of foods that use this additive. You may find some relief for chronic symptoms that have plagued you for years.

FURTHER READINGS

"Carrageenan: How a 'Natural' Food Additive Is Making Us Sick." Cornucopia Institute, Mar. 2013. Accessed Aug. 29, 2019. https://www.cornucopia.org/wp-content/uploads/2013/02/Carrageenan-Report1.pdf

"Carrageenan Market by Type (Kappa, Lota and Lambda), by Application (Food Industry (Dairy, Meat, Beverages and Pet Food), Pharmaceutical Industry and Cosmetics Industry), by Grade (Refined Carrageenan and Semi-refined Carrageenan), by Seaweed Source (Gigartina, Chondrus, Iridaea and Eucheuma) and by Region—Global Growth, Trends, and Forecast to 2024." Market Data Forecast, Oct. 2018. Accessed Aug. 29, 2019. https://www.marketdataforecast.com/market-reports/carrageenan-market

"Carrageenan Market: Growth, Trends and Forecast (2019–2024)." MordorIntelligence.com. Accessed Aug. 29, 2019. https://www.mordorintelligence.com/industry-reports/global-carrageenan-market-industry

"Carrageenan News Update." FoodScienceMatters.com. Accessed Aug. 29, 2019. https://www.foodsciencematters.com/carrageenan.html#poligeenan

"Doubts Surface About Safety of Common Food Additive, Carrageenan." *Chicago Tribune*, Mar. 18, 2013. Accessed Aug. 29, 2019. https://triumphtraining.com/blogs/blog/7559644-carrageenan-concerns-go-mainstream

Fabian, R.J., et al. "Carrageenan-Induced Squamous Metaplasia of the Rectal Mucosa in the Rat." *Gastroenterology*, Aug. 1973, 65(2), 265–276. Accessed Aug. 29, 2019. https://www.researchgate.net/publication/18448524_Carrageenan-Induced_Squamous_Metaplasia_of_the_Rectal_Mucosa_in_the_Rat

"Facts and Figures 2019: US Cancer Death Rate Has Dropped 27% in 25 Years." American Cancer Society, Jan. 8, 2019. Accessed Aug. 30, 2019. https://www.cancer.org/latest-news/facts-and-figures-2019.html

McKim, J.M. "Food Additive Carrageenan: Part 1: A Critical Review of Carrageenan In Vitro Studies, Potential Pitfalls, and Implications for Human Health and Safety."

Critical Review of Toxicology, Mar. 2014, 44(3), 211–243. Accessed Aug. 29, 2019. https://www.ncbi.nlm.nih.gov/pubmed/24456237
"New Study Proves No Adverse Effects of Carrageenan in Human Cells." International Food Additives Council news release, Aug. 10, 2016. Accessed Aug. 30, 2019. https://www.prnewswire.com/news-releases/new-study-proves-no-adverse-effects-of-carrageenan-in-human-cells-300311646.html
Reinagel, Monica. "The Carrageenan Controversy." *Scientific American*, Mar. 19, 2014. Accessed Aug. 30, 2019. https://www.quickanddirtytips.com/health-fitness/healthy-eating/know-your-nutrients/the-carrageenan-controversy
Rustia, Mario, et al. "Lifespan Carcinogenicity Tests with Native Carrageenan in Rats and Hamsters." *Cancer Letters*, Nov. 1980, 11(1), 1–10. Accessed Aug. 29, 2019. https://www.sciencedirect.com/science/article/abs/pii/0304383580901226
Tobacman, J.K. "Review of Harmful Gastrointestinal Effects of Carrageenan in Animal Experiments." *Environmental Health Perspectives*, Oct. 2001, 109(10), 983–984. Accessed Aug. 29, 2019. https://www.ncbi.nlm.nih.gov/pubmed/11675262
Tomarelli, Rudolph M., et al. "Nutritional Quality of Processed Milk Containing Carrageenan." *Journal of Agricultural Food Chemistry*, May 1, 1974, 22(5), 819–824. Accessed Aug. 29, 2019. https://pubs.acs.org/doi/abs/10.1021/jf60195a037

Chocolate

WHAT IS IT?

The fermented, roasted, and ground seeds of the cacao tree produce the basis for the most popular candies in the United States and many countries around the world. Once the seeds are ground, the resulting cocoa mass is heated until liquid, forming a substance called chocolate liquor (though it has no alcohol content) that gets separated into cocoa butter and cocoa solids. These plant-based substances—liquor, butter, and solids—in varying proportions are used to create most of the chocolate we eat.

Chocolate is not naturally sweet; the addition of dairy products and sugar takes the bitter cocoa to the next level in terms of pleasing taste, that satisfying "snap" as we bite into it, and the smooth, creamy mouthfeel consumers love, but this also boosts the calories significantly. Excessive consumption of chocolate plays a role in obesity, which in turn leads to diabetes, heart disease, some cancers, and even Alzheimer's disease.

Chocolate comes to consumers in candy bars, truffles, solid molded shapes, and as a flavoring or mix-in to cookies, cakes, other baked goods, ice cream, mocha and cocoa drinks, and sauces used in some cuisines. Varieties include dark chocolate, which contains between 50 and 90 percent cocoa solids; milk chocolate, which may contain between 10 and 50 percent cocoa solids; and white chocolate, which contains cocoa butter but no solids. More recently, cocoa and dark chocolate have been packaged as "therapeutic" doses with low to no sugar or dairy content.

The growing category of premium-priced chocolate candies ranks chocolate according to the percentage of pure chocolate in the mix, as opposed to sugar, milk, butter, vegetable oil, and other ingredients. A 70-percent chocolate bar, for example, is a very dark chocolate that may taste bitter because of the dominance of pure cocoa over sugar. A Hershey's milk chocolate bar, in contrast, may have just 10 percent chocolate, with sugar, milk, and other ingredients comprising the other 90 percent and giving the bar its characteristic creamy sweetness.

CURRENT CONSUMPTION STATISTICS AND TRENDS

Chocolate is the number one candy consumed in the United States, dominating the confectionary industry with a 75 percent share of the candy market—and its share continues to grow as consumer interest in organic and premium chocolates increases. Sales of chocolate dominate the market at $11.2 billion in the year ended July 15, 2018, according to *Food Business News*. This represents a 0.7 percent increase over 2017. Some $5.3 billion of this extravagant number represents sales of larger items, greater than 3.5 ounces in weight—presumably large bars or bags containing multiple candies and molded chocolates like Easter bunnies. (For reference, the single-serving bag of plain M&Ms® at a checkout counter is 1.69 ounces, while a two-piece Reese's® Peanut Butter Cups package weighs 1.5 ounces.) During the COVID-19 pandemic, the National Confectioners Association reported that sales of chocolate grew 5.5 percent, with much of this in premium chocolate—a niche market that grew by 12.5 percent.

The confectionary industry produces a steady stream of new variations on old favorites to maintain this momentum. M&Ms' coated chocolate candies, for example, only came in plain and peanut varieties for decades, but now include more than thirty varieties, with seasonal flavors like white chocolate candy corn and hot cocoa and specialties like raspberry and crunchy espresso. Dove® chocolate, the premium brand made by Mars Inc., now features more than fifty varieties, from bite-sized squares and bars to fancy truffles and a line of coated ice cream products.

NUTRITIONAL INFORMATION

Cocoa butter contains fat, more than half of which is saturated fat. This has the effect of increasing total cholesterol in the human body by boosting the levels of LDL cholesterol, also known as "bad" cholesterol. Nearly all chocolate products, with the notable exceptions of unsweetened cocoa and baking chocolate, contain considerable amounts of sugar, which are implicated in the development of dental cavities, obesity, high blood pressure, diabetes, and coronary artery disease.

Both cocoa liquor and cocoa butter contain compounds known as flavanols, which are also found in a number of other plant-based foods. The flavanols found in these cocoa products include catechins, which are the only flavanols in chocolate that do not bind to sugar, making them easier for the body to absorb. The more prevalent flavanol in chocolate is epicatechin, which can be classified as an antioxidant and which may have positive effects on human blood circulation and cognitive activity when administered in large doses (more on this later).

Depending on the brand and variety, additional ingredients in chocolate can include some form of lecithin, a thickening agent; vanilla extract (made from vanilla beans) or vanillin, a cheaper alternative made from wood pulp and paper industry by-products; high-fructose corn syrup; corn syrup solids; partially hydrogenated oils that add trans fats; artificial flavors and colors, produced using synthetics; "emulsifiers" that replace some of the pricier cocoa butter; and preservatives like potassium sorbate. Some chocolate candy substitutes sugar alcohols (which are neither sugar nor alcohol and are detailed elsewhere in this book) to reduce or eliminate the overall sugar content.

HISTORY

The first signs of cultivation of cocoa beans appeared in 1500 BC, when the native Olmecs in Mesoamerica, living in what is now south-central Mexico, turned the wild-growing beans into a domestic crop. The Olmecs introduced the Mayan civilization to the beans somewhere around 300 BC; the Mayans ground the beans and made them into an unsweetened drink consumed only by those of the elite class. As the Mayans moved northward from South America into Mesoamerica between AD 600 and 1000, they established cocoa plantations in the Yucatan and used the beans both for consumption and as currency.

In the 1200s, the Maya began to trade with the Aztecs, who drank the bitter cocoa liquid and decided it needed additional flavoring. These creative newcomers to cocoa added cinnamon, pepper, vanilla, and chiles, and the drink quickly gained popularity with the Aztec elite. The Aztecs advanced this exclusivity by restricting the sharing of "cacahuatl" with anyone but the most noble among them and even impose the first tax on cocoa beans. They believe that one of their pantheon of gods, Quetzalcoatl, gave them the beans—and in 1519, when Spanish explorer Hernando Cortez arrived on their shores, they mistook him for Quetzalcoatl and shared the beans with him. As the Aztecs used cocoa beans as money, Cortez saw an opportunity for massive wealth and built a cocoa plantation in Spain's name, conquering the Aztecs within the decade and taking their cocoa beans and chocolate recipes back to the Spanish royal court. King Charles V also realized the opportunity this new food provided, so he assigned the processing of the nation's imported cocoa beans to the monasteries, where it remained a closely guarded secret for nearly a century. Here some wise Spaniard substituted sugar for the chiles and other spices in the traditional drink, turning cocoa into the chocolate we know.

Such a confection could not stay under wraps forever, and in the early 1600s, a traveler from Italy discovered it and brought it home with him. Soon demand in Italy became so great that "cioccolatieri" opened all over the country, and the rich drink's popularity spread throughout Europe. By 1700, chocolate found its way into pastries, and solid bars of chocolate—not the creamily blended kind we know now, but with a grittier texture—became an exciting new treat. Chocolate circled back to the Americas, arriving first in Boston in 1712 as an import from Europe. The turning point, however, came in 1795, when Dr. Joseph Fry used a steam engine to grind cocoa beans, moving the production of chocolate from an artisan activity to a machine-driven enterprise. In 1847, Fry's grandson, Francis, mixed cocoa powder with cocoa butter and discovered that the resulting paste could be molded into figures and bars, and while these still had a grainy texture and lacked the smoothness we now expect from chocolate bars, he nonetheless opened up a new category in the market. Other innovators including the Cadbury brothers in England, Ghirardelli in San Francisco, and Daniel Peter—the neighbor of Henri Nestlé—perfected the process and added their own ingenuity to create new "eating chocolates." The Swiss developed a method known as "conching" to produce a smoother, creamier chocolate, and this modern chocolate became a standard throughout the industry. In 1895, Milton S. Hershey created the first mass-produced chocolate bar that virtually anyone could afford, and he met with such success that he opened his model factory town, Hersheyville, in Pennsylvania just five years later.

Today chocolate reaches every part of the world and is available to anyone, and it features flavors that know no bounds, including some that hearken back to the Aztecs' chile-and-cinnamon concoction. The Ivory Coast in Africa produces the largest share of the world's cocoa beans, while the Netherlands leads the industry in grinding cocoa and exporting it to manufacturers on six continents.

THE CONTROVERSY

Scientists have put considerable effort into attempting to prove that chocolate, especially dark chocolate, may have a beneficial effect on health. This effort may appear on the surface to be driven by humanity's need to justify the massive quantities it consumes of this high-fat, high-sugar confection. The truth, however, is quite different: Most of this research has originated with chocolate manufacturers looking to increase profits in the face of declining sales of milk chocolate, which generally contains more fat and sugar than its dark counterpart.

Many studies about the benefits of flavanols, plant nutrients that appear naturally in cocoa, have been conducted or supported by the research laboratories at Mars Inc., one of the world's largest manufacturers of chocolate and chocolate products. Flavanols are a class of flavonoid, antioxidants that can protect the body's cells from free radicals—substances that form in the normal course of living, but that can damage healthy cells and cause a number of diseases. Mars conducts "the world's largest program studying the dietary effects of cocoa flavonoids," according to the company's website. Obviously, findings that chocolate may be beneficial to health can be of great benefit to the company, though Mars itself cautions, "Before you stock up on chocolate, remember these benefits come from compounds in cocoa pods, little of which can be found in your typical chocolate bar." Mars has conducted or participated in more than 160 studies to date on chocolate's health benefits, including many of the studies published in peer-reviewed scientific journals.

In 2006, a study supported by Mars and conducted at Harvard Medical School and Brigham Women's Hospital in Boston determined that ingestion of cocoa rich in flavanols can have a positive effect on health. Eating specific amounts of cocoa served to improve circulation in older adults by dilating blood vessels, which in turn improved their cognitive function. While the data was preliminary, the researchers noted, "The prospect of increasing cerebral function with cocoa flavanols is extremely promising."

In 2009, the journal *Circulation* published a study that examined an isolated population of Kuna natives living on an island off the coast of Panama. The Kunas consumed ten times more cocoa than their counterparts on the mainland, and while this island population maintained low blood pressure throughout their lives, their relatives in Panama developed normal age-related hypertension. This discrepancy led researcher R. Corti and colleagues to propose that the flavanols in cocoa served to keep blood pressure low.

Many studies attempted to prove this hypothesis, including randomized, double-blind studies that limited the possibility of placebo effect—that is, participants realizing that they were eating chocolate and deliberately or inadvertently skewing the resulting health effects. Others are population-based studies, in which existing data is used to draw conclusions about large groups of people. One of these, conducted in Sweden beginning in 1998, examined how much chocolate (along with ninety-five other foods) more than 33,000 healthy women consumed. Based solely on this survey—which asked these women to recollect a year's worth of chocolate consumption, rather than tracking it as it happened—the Swedish team observed how many of the women had a stroke from 1998 to 2008. They determined that the women who ate the most chocolate had the fewest strokes, leading them to conclude that high chocolate consumption actually protected the women against stroke. The fact that the study was based on memory of past events, providing the researchers with no opportunity to control for hundreds of other variables, reminds us that correlation does not necessarily mean causation.

A series of studies have tested the hypothesis that cocoa's flavanols may interfere with the development of colon cancer. These studies involved *in vitro* (cell cultures in a laboratory) and *in vivo* (tests on animals, usually mice) models, not human beings, and subsequent studies involving humans had mixed result in finding a correlation between cocoa consumption and a reduced risk of colorectal cancer. In fact, a number of studies found that chocolate consumption actually increased the risk of colon cancer in humans, because of the effect of the high refined carbohydrate and sugar intake on insulin and IGF-1, a cancer catalyst.

A 2014 book by neuroscientist Will Clower titled *Eat Chocolate, Lose Weight* recommended that a single square of dark chocolate allowed to melt on the tongue twenty minutes before a meal had the effect of reducing appetite for a meal by as much as half. Despite the very specific limitations Clower detailed in his book for an appropriate use of dark chocolate as an appetite suppressant, the book's title and the resulting media sound bites did not convey this message in its entirety to the public. Instead, chocolate as a weight loss tool became part of the new definition of dark chocolate as a "superfood," supposedly loaded with nutrients and disease-fighting agents that chocolate simply does not contain.

These are just a few of the studies that have led the news media to announce that "Chocolate is good for you!" A 2012 article in the news site *The Daily Beast*, for example, lists eleven ways that chocolate—any chocolate, regardless of flavanol content or grams of sugar—improves health, from decreasing the risk of heart attack and stroke to preventing cancer and diabetes, as well as helping consumers do math and actually making a person lose weight. A 2018 article on the Healthline website calls dark chocolate "one of the best sources of antioxidants on the planet," a claim that is patently false according to virtually every study about chocolate and flavanols.

Based on the previous decade's research examining the health benefits of chocolate, the European Food Safety Authority (EFSA) seemed satisfied that at least some of the claims had merit. In 2013 Barry Callebaut, an ingredients supplier in Europe, won approval from the EFSA of his claim that 2.5 g of dark chocolate per day that contained 200 mg of cocoa flavanols "contributes to normal blood circulation by helping to maintain the elasticity of the blood vessels." Callebaut licensed this claim to the few chocolate manufacturers that could prove their chocolate contained the requisite levels of flavanols, but food scientists at three German universities produced research in 2016 that refuted it. They noted that even the chocolates that could make the case that they had 200 mg of flavanols did not necessarily have 100 mg of epicatechin, the only flavanol in cocoa that actually affects blood pressure. A quantity of cocoa that contains 200 mg of flavanols usually has only about 46 mg of epicatechin, the researchers reported. They, in turn, cited several studies in which quantities of epicatechin lower than 100 mg had no effect on blood pressure.

Some researchers have concluded that certain brands of dark chocolate with high cocoa content do indeed lower participants' blood pressure by a statistically significant 3.1 points (or less). While this may be good news for chocolate lovers, using nothing but dark chocolate to control hypertension would be impractical and ineffective for most people with high blood pressure, as the fat and sugar content contributes to weight gain, which leads to heart disease and diabetes.

The preparation of mass-produced chocolate can have a limiting effect on its health benefits as well. Many products containing cocoa powder or cocoa liquor go through Dutch processing to improve flavor, color, and texture, during which they are mixed with alkali. This makes the chocolate darker (Oreo cookies, e.g., use heavily alkalized chocolate) and reduces its bitterness. Alkali also makes cocoa powder easier to disperse in liquids, so products like instant hot chocolate and unsweetened baking cocoa often have been processed with alkali. In chemical terms, chocolate is highly acidic, and alkalization adds a base to cocoa powder, effectively neutralizing its chemical reaction in baking and cooking. In the United States, products containing alkalized chocolate have to say so on their packaging.

The thing about alkali, however, is that it reduces the amount of flavanols in the chocolate. A 2008 study measured the flavanol content, antioxidation efficiency, and total polyphenol content of cocoa processed without alkali, as well as lightly, medium, and heavily alkalized cocoa. Researcher K.B. Miller and colleagues discovered that natural cocoa had the highest total flavanols at 34.6 ± 6.8 μg/g. This dropped significantly as more alkali was added: The lightly alkalized cocoa retained 13.8 ± 7.3 μg/g, the medium alkalized cocoa had just 7.8 ± 4.0 μg/g, and the heavily alkalized powder measured 3.9 ± 1.8 μg/g of flavanols. As with most processed foods, chocolate becomes less nutritious even as it becomes more flavorful.

So how much is a therapeutic "dose" of dark chocolate? With so many variables affecting the amounts of epicatechin per bar, there is no easy way for the average consumer to judge this. Chocolate bars generally do not have this kind of technical information on the wrapper, so some significant research may be required before we can make the best choice from hundreds of varieties. If chocolate lovers find this a disappointing result of all the promised benefits, keep in mind that other foods have the same flavanol content as an ounce of dark chocolate without the added fat and sugar: tea, cranberries, peanuts, onions, apples, and red wine, for example. Alternately, Mars Inc. has used its research to produce its Cocoa Via line of products, including cocoa extract capsules and premeasured powder packets (to be diluted in water, yogurt, or tea) with 375 mg of flavanols per serving.

Those looking to rationalize their choice of delicious chocolate over other methods of lowering blood pressure and improving overall health—such as diet and exercise—may find that their favorite treat does not provide the therapeutic benefits they were hoping to obtain. As the adage goes, "If it looks too good to be true, it probably is."

FURTHER READINGS

"A Chocolate Timeline: Follow One of Man's Favorite Foods." *The Nibble*, May 2010. Accessed May 21, 2019. https://www.thenibble.com/reviews/main/chocolate/the-history-of-chocolate.asp

Bonetti, Francesco, et al. "Nootropics, Functional Foods and Dietary Patterns for Prevention of Cognitive Decline." *Nutritional and Functional Foods for Healthy Aging*, Watson, Ronald Ross, ed. London, UK: Academic Press, Elsevier, 2017. Accessed May 20, 2019. https://www.sciencedirect.com/topics/pharmacology-toxicology-and-pharmaceutical-science/flavanols

EFSA Panel on Dietetic Products, Nutrition and Allergies. "Scientific Opinion on the Modification of the Authorisation of a Health Claim Related to Cocoa Flavanols and

Maintenance of Normal Endothelium-Dependent Vasodilation Pursuant to Article 13(5) of Regulation (EC) No 1924/2006 Following a Request in Accordance with Article 19 of Regulation (EC) No 1924/2006." *EFSA Journal*, May 5, 2014. Accessed May 25, 2019. https://efsa.onlinelibrary.wiley.com/doi/10.2903/j.efsa.2014.3654

Egan, Brent M., et al. "Does Dark Chocolate Have a Roll in the Prevention and Management of Hypertension? Commentary on the Evidence." *Hypertension*, June 2010, 56(6). Accessed May 22, 2019. https://www.ahajournals.org/doi/full/10.1161/HYPERTENSIONAHA.110.151522

Fisher, Naomi D.L., et al. "Cocoa Flavanols and Brain Perfusion." *Journal of Cardiovascular Pharmacology*, June 2006, 47, S210–S214. Accessed May 25, 2019. https://journals.lww.com/cardiovascularpharm/Fulltext/2006/06001/Cocoa_Flavanols_and_Brain_Perfusion.17.aspx

Gunnars, Kris. "7 Proven Health Benefits of Dark Chocolate." Healthline, June 25, 2018. Accessed May 25, 2019. https://www.healthline.com/nutrition/7-health-benefits-dark-chocolate

"Heart Healthy Benefits of Chocolate." Cleveland Clinic. Accessed May 22, 2019. https://my.clevelandclinic.org/health/articles/16774-heart-healthy-benefits-of-chocolate

Heller, Jake. "11 Reasons Chocolate's Good For You." *The Daily Beast*, Mar. 28, 2012. Accessed May 25, 2019. https://www.thedailybeast.com/11-reasons-chocolates-good-for-you

Larsson, Susanna C., et al. "Chocolate Consumption and Risk of Stroke in Women." *Journal of the American College of Cardiology*, Oct. 18, 2011, 58(17), 1828–1829. Accessed May 25, 2019. https://www.sciencedirect.com/science/article/pii/S0735109711028440?via%3Dihub

Latif, R. "Chocolate/Cocoa and Human Health: A Review." *Netherlands Journal of Medicine*, Mar. 2013, 71(2), 63–68. Accessed May 20, 2019. http://www.njmonline.nl/getpdf.php?id=1269

Martin, Maria Angeles, et al. "Preventive Effects of Cocoa and Cocoa Antioxidants on Colon Cancer." *Diseases*, Mar. 2016, 4(1). Accessed May 26, 2019. https://www.ncbi.nlm.nih.gov/pmc/articles/PMC5456306/

Miller, K.B., et al. "Impact of Alkalization on the Antioxidant and Flavanol Content of Commercial Cocoa Powders." *Journal of Agricultural and Food Chemistry*, Sept. 24, 2008, 56(18), 8527–8533. Accessed May 21, 2019. https://www.ncbi.nlm.nih.gov/pubmed/18710243

Nieburg, Oliver. "Healthy Chocolate: EU Cocoa Flavanol Health Claim 'Should Be Revised,' Say Researchers." *Confectionary News*, July 5, 2016. Accessed May 22, 2019. https://www.confectionerynews.com/Article/2016/07/06/EU-cocoa-flavanol-health-claim-should-be-revised-Study

"North America Confectionery Market—Segmented by Product Type, Distribution Channel and Geography—Growth, Trends, and Forecast (2018–2023)." Research and Markets, May 2018. Accessed May 20, 2019. https://www.researchandmarkets.com/research/74brv3/the_north_america?w=4

Watrous, Monica. "State of the Industry: Confectionary." *Food Business News*, Dec. 17, 2018. Accessed May 20, 2019. https://www.foodbusinessnews.net/articles/12971-state-of-the-industry-confectionery

Watrous, Monica. "State of the Industry: Confectionary." *Food Business News*, Dec. 15, 2020. Accessed April 13, 2021. https://www.foodbusinessnews.net/articles/17383-confectionery-industry-boosted-by-low-sugar-innovation

Coconut Oil

WHAT IS IT?

Coconut oil comes from the flesh of the coconut. Products fall into two general categories: refined and unrefined or virgin.

Refined varieties are extracted from the dried coconut meat (also known as copra) and usually have no odor or taste. This is because the refined versions have been processed more aggressively, filtered to remove any impurities, and treated to lighten their color or to remove coconut scent and flavor. Chemicals including hexane may be required to help extract the oil from the coconut meat.

"Virgin" or unrefined coconut oil is pressed from the fresh coconut meat and may retain more coconut aroma and taste than refined versions. Virgin varieties contain no added chemicals.

Oils cannot be considered "whole" foods, as the very definition of oil dictates that it be extracted from plant material. Some coconut oils have been labeled "whole kernel" by their manufacturers, a moniker that indicates that the brown inside skin of the coconut remained on the nut meat during the oil extraction process. Whole kernel oils retain more flavor and nutrients, making them preferable in some applications, while some consumers prefer the appearance and gentler scent of white kernel coconut oil, the product of coconuts with the inside skin removed.

Most brands extract coconut oil using the expeller-pressed or cold-pressed methods. Expeller pressing uses a machine at high pressure to extract the oil from the meat and usually involves heating the meat to 120°F or above. Cold-pressed coconut oil uses the same process but without the heat and may allow the oil to retain more of its nutrients. A third process, centrifuging, begins with removal of the coconut milk from the meat and then involves removal of the shell and spinning the meat in a centrifuge, crushing the remaining meat to a fine paste. This process separates the meat from the oil remaining in it. The many steps and specialized machinery involved make this a particularly expensive process, so centrifuged coconut oil tends to be pricier than expeller-pressed or cold-pressed varieties.

Coconut oil can be used in cooking (though at relatively low temperatures—it will begin to smoke between 350°F and 400°F), but its high saturated fat content requires that its use as a cooking oil be limited as part of a healthy diet. Based on its flavor, its high saturated fat content, and its overall popularity with consumers, many snack manufacturers use coconut oil in products including cookies, cakes, cupcakes, ice cream, and yogurt. The cosmetics industry has embraced its power as a frizz smoother, lubricant, and moisturizer, adding it to all kinds of skin and hair care products, from facial masks to high-end creams and conditioners.

CURRENT CONSUMPTION STATISTICS AND TRENDS

The firm Market Research Future reported in May 2019 that the coconut oil market is expected to reach $8.4 billion by 2025. According to MarketWatch, the global market for virgin coconut oil (VCO) alone reached $650 million in 2018 and is expected to continue to grow at 2.3 percent annually through 2025.

The U.S. consumption hit a peak in 2009 with 598,000 megatons sold, according to the U.S. Department of Agriculture, but it declined nearly 19 percent the following year. In recent years, consumption has dropped to about 445,000 megatons. Coconut oil has lost some of its luster as the American Heart Association (AHA) issued a presidential advisory in 2017 to avoid saturated fat—coconut oil is up to 90 percent saturated fat—and replace it with polyunsaturated vegetable oil. Other studies suggest that there is not enough evidence to conclude that saturated fat provides a direct route to heart disease or that eliminating it entirely will protect against heart problems. (See Saturated Fat later in this book.)

NUTRITIONAL INFORMATION

Coconut oil is a particularly fatty fat, surpassing palm kernel oil at 82 percent saturated fat, according to the AHA report. Some reports say that coconut oil's saturated fat content is as high as 90 percent. This is the highest saturated fat content of any of the commonly used oils, a fact that led the AHA to recommend that it be decreased in any healthy diet.

The rest of coconut oil's composition is small amounts of polyunsaturated and monounsaturated fat, the part considered "good" fat (or at least not harmful fat). Together, they add up to 100 percent fat, a good reminder that coconut oil is purely fat.

The oil does not contain any cholesterol, though it plays a role in creating LDL cholesterol in people who consume it. Tiny amounts of vitamins may be present in some products, but they are not enough to make it to the nutrition facts label.

Some versions of refined coconut oil may contain partially hydrogenated unsaturated fats, a processed ingredient that acts as a preservative and keeps solidified oil from melting in a warm environment. Partially hydrogenated fats are trans fats, the most destructive fats to the human body. Read the label before purchasing any coconut oil to be sure that it does not contain these harmful ingredients.

HISTORY

References to the fruit that would eventually be named the coconut can be found in texts dating back to the fifth century AD. Use of the oil extracted from the skin and meat predates recorded history, beginning to appear in the journals of explorers and in stories from far eastern and southern Asia in the ninth century. People who had access to the oil used it as an aid to healing wounds, as a massage oil for sore muscles, in making candles, and as a skin lotion and hair restorative. Pacific island dwellers believed the oil could protect against illness, cure ailments, encourage bone growth, and clear up acne.

A tree of tropical climates, the coconut palm became a cultivated crop in India, Sri Lanka, the Philippines, Malaysia, Indonesia, and Papua New Guinea at least two thousand years ago. Its white flesh served as a food staple, and the water or "milk" that naturally resides inside provided additional nourishment and food flavoring. The large fruit had many names before the 1700s, when the Portuguese finally labeled it "coco," using their language's word for head.

In the late 1800s, European businesses saw value in coconut oil as a product, because of its versatility as an ingredient in soap and as a cooking aid. They used their land holdings in Southeast Asia, the southern Pacific islands, and the Caribbean islands to build plantations for coconut production, creating a new market in Europe and the United States for the exotic oil. The arrival of World War II put an end to this trade temporarily, curtailing the availability of this as well as a number of other oils pressed from tropical plants. (This turned out to be a lucky break for soy-based oils, as soybeans could be grown in cooler, drier climates like the American Great Plains.)

When the war ended, soybean and vegetable oils had replaced coconut, palm, and olive oil in cooking, and while coconut oil producers scrambled to get back the market share they'd lost, they met with a new obstacle: the science of saturated fat. In the 1950s, Ancel Keys, a well-known nutrition scientist, determined that too much saturated fat in the human diet correlated directly with high cholesterol levels. Other researchers tested this hypothesis and found a direct link between saturated fat and cholesterol, though these findings were disputed by coconut oil producers. People in the south seas who had used coconut oil in cooking for centuries did not develop this high cholesterol, they said, because they also ate plenty of fish rich in omega-3 fatty acids. The combination of coconut oil and fish actually produced better health, they claimed. The research that coconut oil producers questioned may also have involved hydrogenated oil, which is loaded with trans fats—so these additional, destructive fats may have been the actual culprit that caused the spikes in cholesterol.

This early research and a number of more recent studies have kept the question open of whether coconut oil has a healthful or health-damaging effect. The now decades-old controversy has not reached a definitive conclusion, but coconut oil has come to the fore as a key wellness ingredient among those looking for naturopathic remedies for common ailments. Most of these people cite studies that indicate that elements of coconut oil—lauric acid in particular—have a beneficial effect against a range of diseases, from osteoporosis to colon cancer.

THE CONTROVERSY

The multibillion-dollar coconut oil industry has done a remarkable job of marketing its products as healthy, so much so that in a recent survey, 72 percent of Americans called coconut oil a "healthy" food, while only 37 percent of nutritionists agreed. This achievement may delight shareholders, but it flies in the face of careful research completed as far back as 1995, when a team at the Department of Human Nutrition at the University of Otago in New Zealand compared the effects of coconut oil, butter, and safflower oil in a small cohort of twenty-eight people with slightly elevated cholesterol. The subjects all followed the same diets for six weeks at a time, first using coconut oil as the primary fat, then butter, and finally safflower oil. The researchers found that butter elevated LDL cholesterol significantly, and coconut oil came in a very close second. Safflower oil did not elevate the subjects' total or LDL cholesterol.

The T.H. Chan School of Public Health at Harvard University provides information that helps us understand the difference between manufacturers' marketing claims and research results. Saturated fats can be sorted into three distinct types: short-, medium- (MCTs), and long-chain triglycerides (LCTs; fatty acids). LCTs get stored in the body's fat tissue, often taking up residence and increasing body weight. MCTs, however, go to the liver, where they are quickly metabolized so the body can use them for energy. Studies using a special formulation of coconut oil high in MCTs determined that the coconut oil could promote a feeling of fullness sooner in a meal and that it did not get stored as fat in the body. This formulation, however, is not the coconut oil sold in stores as food. The coconut oil in supermarkets contains lauric acid as its predominant saturated fat; lauric acid sometimes acts like a long-chain fatty acid and gets stored in the body's fat cells and sometimes acts like an MCT and gets converted to energy. VCO also contains capric and caprylic acids, two additional MCTs, but in much smaller amounts than lauric acid. These, accompanied by smaller amounts of myristic and palmitic triglycerides (which are long chain), make up virtually all of the fat in coconut oil. "It's important not to draw conclusions about the benefits of coconut oil based on studies with oils called medium-chain triglyceride (MCT) oil," the Mayo Clinic warns.

This has not stopped coconut oil manufacturers from claiming that their products can assist in weight loss, based on the action of MCTs in experiments with this manipulated oil. These claims are based on studies that tested MCTs, not coconut oil specifically (in fact, coconut oil is not mentioned in the studies), and found that men who consumed more MCTs than LCTs expended more energy and lost more fat tissue than those who ate LCTs (St-Onge, 2003; Dulloo, 1996).

One of the lead researchers on such a study, Marie-Pierre St-Onge, PhD, at Columbia University, was quick to make this clarification in the popular press. "There's strong data on the weight loss properties of MCT oil in general, but not as much for coconut oil specifically," she explained to a writer at *Woman's Day*. "Coconut oil is only 13.5 percent of purified MCT. To get 10g [grams] of MCT, you need to eat 80g coconut oil. 80g of any oil in a single day is a lot of oil, especially coconut oil, which is so high in saturated fat" (Natale and Lee, 2019).

Small studies have borne out this conflict between consuming enough coconut oil to have an impact on weight loss and maintaining a heart-healthy diet. A 2017 study involving thirty-two volunteers in Thailand had each of the participants take 15 mL of VCO twice daily (a total of 26 g of saturated fat) or the same amount of a control solution for eight weeks. At the end of the trial, the participants who had taken VCO saw an increase in HDL (good) cholesterol. "Daily consumption of 30 mL VCO in young healthy adults significantly increased high-density lipoprotein cholesterol," the researchers reported in *Evidence-Based Complementary Alternative Medicine* (Chinwong et al., 2017). The short-term study did not delve into the potential issues created by ingesting so much saturated fat on a daily basis, however; the AHA recommends no more than 13 g of saturated fat each day or about 5 percent of a person's total caloric intake.

A 2009 study on forty women with abdominal obesity placed these women on a strict diet and an exercise program that involved walking for fifty minutes daily and also gave them supplements containing either 30 mL of coconut oil or soybean oil. The group that received coconut oil lost more belly fat and saw an increase in HDL, while both groups experienced some weight loss.

So far, all of the studies conducted on coconut oil have been short term and with small groups of people, and they have incorporated coconut oil into a larger and more comprehensive diet and exercise program. The result? "There is no evidence that coconut oil will have a beneficial effect on weight loss if you simply add it to your diet," the Mayo Clinic reports. Much more comprehensive, long-term research will be required to understand if this oil, with its sky-high saturated fat content, may actually have a positive effect on the human body.

A detailed review of studies to date on coconut oil's effects on weight loss, heart disease, and other illnesses appeared in *Nutrition Bulletin* in 2016. The authors note:

> Recipe books, advertisements and some journal articles are claiming that coconut oil is a cure-all product that has weight reduction, cholesterol-lowering, wound healing and immune system, energy and memory-boosting effects and can be used to treat Crohn's disease, irritable bowel syndrome, thyroid conditions, diabetes, and well as Alzheimer's and Parkinson's diseases.

After a careful enumeration of the studies to date and their relative credibility, the paper concludes,

> Due to existing knowledge regarding saturated fatty acids and heart disease, evidence . . . suggesting that coconut oil raises plasma lipids and a lack of large, well-controlled human studies published in peer-reviewed journals demonstrating clear health benefits of coconut oil, frequent use of coconut oil should not be advised.
>
> (Lockyer and Stanner, 2016)

In 2017, the journal *Cell Death Discovery* published a study that indicates that lauric acid may prompt the death of colon, endometrial, and breast cancer cells. "Collectively, our findings may pave the way to better understand the anticancer action of [lauric acid], although additional studies are warranted to further corroborate its usefulness in more comprehensive therapeutic approaches," the researchers concluded (Lappano et al., 2017).

Until such long-term controlled studies emerge, coconut oil's most effective uses continue to be topical, as an aid to complexion and a conditioner to restore damaged hair. If it does have an effect against any disease, much more research will be required to determine the delivery method, dosage, and other protocols that may be involved in using components of coconut oil in treatment. Simply eating more of it is not medically significant against cancer or any other illness.

FURTHER READINGS

Assunção, Monica L., et al. "Effects of Dietary Coconut Oil on the Biochemical and Anthropometric Profiles of Women Presenting Abdominal Obesity." *Lipids*, July 2009, 44(7), 593–601. Accessed Sept. 3, 2019. https://link.springer.com/article/10.1007/s11745-009-3306-6

Chinwong, Surarong, et al. "Daily Consumption of Virgin Coconut Oil Increases High-Density Lipoprotein Cholesterol Levels in Health Volunteers: A Randomized Crossover Trial." *Evidence-Based Complementary Alternative Medicine*, Dec. 4, 2017. Accessed Sept. 3, 2019. https://www.ncbi.nlm.nih.gov/pmc/articles/PMC5745680/

"Coconut Oil for Weight Loss: Does It Work?" Mayo Clinic. Accessed Sept. 3, 2019. https://www.mayoclinic.org/healthy-lifestyle/weight-loss/in-depth/coconut-oil-and-weight-loss/art-20450177

"Coconut Oil Market Research Report-Global Forecast Till 2025." Market Research Future, Feb. 2019. Accessed Sept. 3, 2019. https://www.marketresearchfuture.com/reports/coconut-oil-market-7452

Cox, C., et al. "Effects of Coconut Oil, Butter, and Safflower Oil on Lipids and Lipoproteins in Persons with Moderately Elevated Cholesterol Levels." *Journal of Lipid Research*, Aug. 1995, 36(8), 1787–1795. Accessed Sept. 3, 2019. https://www.ncbi.nlm.nih.gov/pubmed/7595099?dopt=Abstract

Dulloo, A.G; Fathi, M.; Mensi, N.; and Girandier, L. "Twenty-Four-Hour Energy Expenditure and Urinary Catecholamines of Humans Consuming Low-to-Moderate Amounts of Medium-Chain Triglycerides: A Dose-Response Study in a Human Respiratory Chamber." *European Journal of Clinical Nutrition*, Mar. 1996, 50(3), 152–158. Accessed Sept. 3, 2019. https://www.ncbi.nlm.nih.gov/pubmed/8654328

Lappano, Rosamaria, et al. "The Lauric Acid-Activated Signaling Prompts Apoptosis in Cancer Cells." *Cell Death Discovery*, 2017, 3, 17063. Accessed Sept. 4, 2019. https://www.ncbi.nlm.nih.gov/pmc/articles/PMC5601385/

Lockyer, S.; and Stanner, S., "Coconut Oil—A Nutty Idea?" Facts Behind the Headlines, *Nutrition Bulletin*, Feb. 16, 2016. Accessed Sept. 4, 2019. https://onlinelibrary.wiley.com/doi/full/10.1111/nbu.12188

Natale, Nicol; and Lee, Byron P. "Can Coconut Oil Help with Weight Loss? Experts Break It Down." Woman's Day, Feb. 8, 2019. Accessed Sept. 3, 2019. https://www.womansday.com/health-fitness/a58976/coconut-oil-weight-loss/

"The Nutrition Source: Coconut Oil." T.H. Chan School of Public Health, Harvard University. Accessed Sept. 3, 2019. https://www.hsph.harvard.edu/nutritionsource/food-features/coconut-oil/

Quealy, K.; and Sanger-Katz, M. "Is Sushi 'Healthy'? What About Granola? Where Americans and Nutritionists Disagree." *New York Times*, July 5, 2016. Accessed Sept. 3, 2019. https://www.nytimes.com/interactive/2016/07/05/upshot/is-sushi-healthy-what-about-granola-where-americans-and-nutritionists-disagree.html?_r=0%20Y.

Sacks, Frank M., et al. "Dietary Fats and Cardiovascular Disease: A Presidential Advisory From the American Heart Association." *Circulation*, June 15, 2017, 136(3). Accessed Sept. 3, 2019. https://www.ahajournals.org/doi/full/10.1161/CIR.0000000000000510

St-Onge, M.P.; and Jones, P.J. "Greater Rise in Fat Oxidation with Medium-Chain Triglyceride Consumption Relative to Long-Chain Triglyceride Is Associated with Lower Initial Body Weight and Greater Loss of Subcutaneous Adipose Tissue." *International Journal of Obesity and Related Metabolic Disorders*, Dec. 2003, 27(12), 1565–1571. Accessed Sept. 3, 2019. https://www.ncbi.nlm.nih.gov/pubmed/12975635

"Understanding Coconut Oil." Kimberton Whole Foods. Accessed Sept. 3, 2019. https://www.kimbertonwholefoods.com/decoding-coconut-oil/#.XW6qOC3MwWo

"United States Coconut Oil Domestic Consumption by Year." IndexMundi. Accessed Sept. 3, 2019. https://www.indexmundi.com/agriculture/?country=us&commodity=coconut-oil&graph=domestic-consumption

"Virgin Coconut Oil Market Size 2019, Global Trends, Industry Share, Growth Drivers, Business Opportunities and Demand Forecast to 2025." MarketWatch, Apr. 3, 2019. Accessed Sept. 3, 2019. https://www.marketwatch.com/press-release/virgin-coconut-oil-market-size-2019-global-trends-industry-share-growth-drivers-business-opportunities-and-demand-forecast-to-2025-2019-04-03

Cruciferous Vegetables

WHAT ARE THEY?

Plants in the family Cruciferae are part of the large category of cruciferous vegetables. Generally, these include leafy greens like arugula, bok choy, broccoli, broccoli rabe, Brussels sprouts, cabbage, cauliflower, Chinese broccoli, Chinese cabbage, collard greens, daikon, garden cress, horseradish, kale, kohlrabi, komatsuna, mizuna, mustard leaves, radish, rutabaga, tatsoi, turnip roots and greens, wasabi, and watercress.

CURRENT CONSUMPTION STATISTICS AND TRENDS

In 2017, the last year for which statistics are available, the world produced 71.45 million metric tons of cabbages and other leafy green vegetables in the cruciferous category. In addition, farms produced twenty-six million metric tons of cauliflower and broccoli. Cruciferous vegetables represented a $13.84 billion market in the United States alone in 2017. California surpasses all other states in fresh vegetable output, according to the USDA, accounting for 60 percent of vegetable production in the country.

As large a market as this is, however, the U.S. growers have seen a decline in the fresh vegetable market in 2018 and 2019, down 9 percent in 2018 alone. Much of this comes from planting less acreage and smaller harvests, in part because of record heat throughout the growing season. *Vegetable Growers News* reported that the decline in production coincides with lower monthly rainfall and higher temperatures, both of which can be attributed to climate change. The difficulty in using the complicated H-2A guest agricultural work program, which allows immigrants to enter the country temporarily to work on industrial farms, also has hindered farms' ability to harvest crops in a timely manner.

While vegetable production fell in 2017 to its lowest point in seventeen years, consumer demand remains high—even in the face of outbreaks of foodborne illness found in leafy green vegetables (specifically romaine, which is not in the cruciferous family). Bagged salads, packaging of pre-cut fresh vegetables, and microwaveable bags of vegetables have spurred purchase rates, even though these convenience products are more expensive. The growth in organic vegetable availability has also influenced the demand.

NUTRITIONAL INFORMATION

These vegetables earn their "superfoods" title for good reason: They are packed with vitamins and minerals the human body needs to function properly. One three-fourth-cup serving of broccoli, for example, contains more than 20 percent of the recommended daily amount of folate, the B vitamin required for cell division and the production of DNA. It also provides plenty of vitamin C, which may protect cells from cancer-causing free radicals and strengthens the immune system. Leafy greens and broccoli supply the body with vitamin K, which we require for blood clotting and bone growth; and broccoli provides potassium, a key element in maintaining a healthy blood pressure. These vegetables also contain glucosinolates, the compounds that give them their bitter taste when chopped, processed, or chewed; glucosinolates, in turn, contain isothiocyanates, which have been found to keep cancer cells from dividing and actively kill tumor cells in the bladder, breast, colon, liver, lung, and stomach of laboratory rats.

Some vegetables in this family provide beta-carotene, which converts into the cognition-boosting vitamin A, while others have antioxidants including anthocyanins, agents that fight heart disease by promoting blood sugar metabolism and lowering cholesterol levels. Polyphenols, compounds that may lower blood sugar, soothe digestion, and increase brain function, are found in some cruciferous varieties.

In addition, cruciferous vegetables provide plenty of fiber, a key factor in decreasing the risk of colorectal cancer, type 2 diabetes, and coronary artery disease.

HISTORY

Who was the first to determine that cruciferous vegetables are edible? The identity of this person has long since been lost to history, but we can guess that this discovery took place tens of thousands of years ago as the earliest humans sampled wild plants. The first vegetables to be grown domestically may have been cabbages, which appeared in the European countries more than three thousand years ago and in China a millennium before that. The Celts may have been the first to cultivate the leafy plants in Europe, while Egyptians did not begin to grow them until about 300 BC. The name of the brassica family comes from the Roman empire; the inclusion of the vegetable in the writings of Theophrastus, the recognized "father of botany," tells us that cabbage had become a staple in the ancient cities. Cabbage also had medicinal properties, according to the Romans, who ate it before a night of heavy drinking to ease the effects of alcohol and who used the leaves to relieve gout and headaches.

Cultivation of cabbage spread both eastward and westward from Europe, with the first round-headed cabbages showing up in the New World in the fifteenth century at the hands of French explorer Jacques Cartier. By this time, doctors on long ocean voyages used cabbage soaked in brine—a precursor to sauerkraut—as a poultice to treat sailors' wounds and as a food staple to prevent scurvy. European explorers introduced cabbage to China and India, where the easy-to-grow crop quickly became a staple. Today China is the largest producer of cabbage in the world.

Broccoli never grew wild in ancient fields. Cultivated by selective breeding of wild cabbage in the days of the Roman Empire, it originated in the Mediterranean region, where farmers selected the healthiest and tastiest plants from their cabbage crops and bred only those from one year to the next. Eventually, they achieved a plant with tight green flowers and a mild flavor, the ancestor to the broccoli we enjoy today. This process also produced cauliflower, kale, Brussels sprouts, and the attractive red and green cabbage heads preferred by shoppers. Traders and explorers brought these cultivated vegetables to the rest of Europe and to America in the 1700s.

THE CONTROVERSY

While many foods get sporadic and often misplaced credit for fighting or even curing cancer, cruciferous vegetables actually contain glucosinolates and derivatives that result from digestion of these vegetables: sulforaphane and indole-3-carbinol, which have been shown to reduce the risk of bladder, breast, colorectal, endometrial, gastric, lung, ovarian, pancreatic, prostate, and renal cancer. In 2004, a report by the U.S. Department of Agriculture reviewed the epidemiological studies involving these vegetables and concluded that "consumption of cruciferous vegetables protects against cancer more effectively than the total intake of fruits and vegetables" (Keck and Finley). The report explained that this particular family of veggies can affect estrogen metabolism and decrease the activation of carcinogens in the body by inhibiting certain enzymes involved in tumor growth. Cruciferous vegetables also reduce inflammation in the body, making them an excellent choice for people with rheumatoid arthritis, asthma, ulcerative colitis, and other chronic conditions triggered by inflammation.

The National Cancer Institute's review of the many studies linking cruciferous vegetables with lowered cancer risk drew mixed conclusions, however. The institute acknowledges that one study does seem to draw a connection between women who ate more than five servings of these vegetables per week and a lower risk of lung cancer. Another indicates that women (but not men) who consumed a lot of cruciferous vegetables per week had a lower risk of colon cancer. One study compared men who had prostate cancer and men who did not and determined that men who ate more of these vegetables were less likely to have this cancer. Other studies in their review, however, did not deliver a close association between vegetable intake and cancer risk. The institute notes that studies show that these vegetables can have a positive effect on the biomarkers (DNA) of processes in the body that lead to cancer: In one study, indole-3-carbinol "was more effective than placebo" in inhibiting the growth of cancerous cells on the cervix.

The American Institute for Cancer Research tells us that vitamins and minerals ingested by eating food are stronger cancer-fighting agents than supplements made in laboratories, but sales of supplements that claim to contain "cruciferous vegetable extract" or "activated broccoli seed extract" have reached all-time highs as consumers turn to mega-dose pills, many of which are frighteningly expensive. As is the case with many supplements, extracts of broccoli and others in this vegetable family may be much less effective than eating the plant itself, as glucosinolates have to go through the process of digestion to become absorbable in the gastrointestinal tract. In addition, labels on supplements usually do not identify the part of the plant from which the compound has been extracted; glucosinolates in the leaves and florets, for example, are different from those found in the stems and roots.

Why not just eat more vegetables, instead of turning supplements into expensive urine? Some consumers may object to the production of intestinal gas that comes from eating these plants. In general, however, it seems that people will do just about anything to avoid having to eat broccoli, cauliflower, and kale, even though they are cheaper, more nourishing, and more effective solutions to fighting diseases than any packaged supplement.

There is a flip side to this coin, however. Some studies have found that cruciferous vegetables may play a role in hypothyroidism, a condition in which the thyroid does not produce enough hormones. Eaten raw, these vegetables release compounds in the digestive system called goitrogens, which seem to interfere with the body's ability to synthesize thyroid hormones. Some glucosinolates cause the release of thiocyanate ions, which fight iodine in the body and prevent the thyroid gland from functioning properly. This effect has only been produced in animals to date and only with consumption of very large amounts of cruciferous vegetables. In humans, this issue appears only in people who have an iodine deficiency; people who are otherwise healthy do not see an onset of hypothyroidism from eating these vegetables on a daily basis.

With this in mind, the 2015–2020 *Dietary Guidelines for Americans* say that eating two and a half cups of vegetables daily from a variety of subgroups—from dark green, leafy vegetables to starchy ones and legumes—is a healthy choice within a 2,000-calorie-per-day diet. Among these, up to two and a half cups per week of dark green vegetables, including the cruciferous varieties, provides the desired health benefits with no real danger of upsetting a healthy thyroid.

Recently, another issue has come to the surface, this one involving the mineral thallium. It began in 2012 with the work of Ernie Hubbard, a doctor and molecular biologist in Marin County, California, in which he discovered that a select group of his patients had high levels of thallium and cesium in their urine, eliminated through use of a "chelation" process (use of a formulated stimulant to release supposed toxins from the body). He discovered a study published in 2006 in which researchers planted kale, a "hyperaccumulator" of thallium, to draw the mineral from the ground where it had leached from a neighboring industrial site. Hubbard connected the dots and decided that the symptoms his patients showed—fatigue, arrhythmias, gluten sensitivity, mental "fogginess," and hair loss—were all attributable to the amount of thallium they consumed through the large amounts of kale and cabbage they ate on a daily basis.

Here are some of the issues other researchers have found with this theory. First, for kale to contain thallium (or other potentially toxic metal), it must grow in fields where there is thallium in the soil. This is not necessarily a common occurrence, despite the coverage this theory received in the mass media when *Craftsmanship*, an architectural magazine (not, notably, a peer-reviewed medical journal), broke the story in 2015. The media that picked up the story's basic message—that kale may be bad for us because it draws dangerous metals right out of the ground and inserts them into our smoothies and salads—ran with it as if it were an FDA regulation. The fact is that Hubbard's research took place largely in a lab he created for himself in his own kitchen, on the houseboat where he lives, on a carefully selected group of patients. He told the writer at *Craftsmanship* that when he instructed these patients to stop eating so much kale and to use a chelation solution to evacuate any metals in their bodies through their urine, the urine he tested revealed high concentrations of metals including thallium, cesium, nickel, lead, aluminum, and arsenic. He also sent kale samples to a lab and found that they, too, contained this range of metals.

Whether the patients actually got these metals in their systems from kale and cabbage or from any number of other sources (Hubbard tested some jars of baby food and found the metals in there as well), Hubbard's research could not determine for certain. Even the suggestion that kale might be unhealthy, however, set off a storm of media attention with headlines like "Eating Kale Is Making People Seriously Sick" (Delish.com), "Where Is All The Toxic Kale Coming From?" (HealthNewsReview), "Is Kale a Killer?" (DrWell.com), "Eating Too Much Kale May Result in Thallium Poisoning" (FirstWeFeast.com), and "Sorry, Foodies: We're About to Ruin Kale," from the normally more discerning *Mother Jones*.

The fact is that no peer-reviewed journal has published any research on thallium levels in kale and their potential link to any kind of illness. Hubbard's research never rose to the level of peer review.

Thallium is a known toxin to humans, as reported by the Environmental Protection Agency, but the EPA's 2009 report does not suggest that any specific food could carry enough thallium to cause a damaging level of toxicity. The research cited by the EPA does note that hair loss, neurological effects (fatigue, back pain, weakness, inability to walk, and mental effects), and kidney and liver damage all can be caused by thallium, as well as low birth weight in newborns whose mothers are exposed. None of this is associated in any scientific way with consumption of kale or any other cruciferous vegetable, however—the EPA's analysis comes from studies involving rodents and high doses of thallium and related compounds or humans living within close proximity of an industrial site where thallium enters the air and the water supply.

In short, there is no good science that indicates that kale is bad for humans because of its mineral content.

FURTHER READINGS

"AICR's Foods That Fight Cancer: Cruciferous Vegetables." American Institute for Cancer Research. Accessed Sept. 5, 2019. https://www.aicr.org/foods-that-fight-cancer/broccoli-cruciferous.html

Cook, Roberta. "Consumer Fresh Produce Demand Trends." University of California, Davis, June 17, 2016. Accessed Sept. 4, 2019. https://arefiles.ucdavis.edu/uploads/filer_public/53/73/53730f77-1c54-4770-8792-3045e8bc74d2/shtcsecookconsumer20160728.pdf

"Cruciferous Vegetables and Cancer Prevention." National Cancer Institute, June 7, 2012. Accessed Sept. 6, 2019. https://www.cancer.gov/about-cancer/causes-prevention/risk/diet/cruciferous-vegetables-fact-sheet#is-there-evidence-that-cruciferous-vegetables-can-help-reduce-cancer-risk-in-people

Delarge, Barbara, et al. "Cruciferous Vegetables." Linus Pauling Institute Micronutrient Information Center, Oregon State University, Dec. 2016. Accessed Sept. 6, 2019. https://lpi.oregonstate.edu/mic/food-beverages/cruciferous-vegetables

Fenwick, G.R.; Heaney, R.K.; and Mullin, W.J. "Glucosinolates and Their Breakdown Products in Food and Food Plants." *Critical Review of Food Science and Nutrition*, 1983;18(2), 123–201. Accessed Sept. 6, 2019. https://www.ncbi.nlm.nih.gov/pubmed/6337782

Fuentes, Francisco, et al. "Dietary Glucosinolates Sulforaphane, Phenethyl Isothiocyanate, Indole-3-Carbinol/3,3′-Diindolylmethane: Anti-oxidative Stress/Inflammation, Nrf2, Epigenetics/Epigenomics and In Vivo Cancer Chemopreventive Efficacy." *Current Pharmacology Reports*, May 2015, 1(3), 179–196. Accessed Sept. 6, 2019. https://www.ncbi.nlm.nih.gov/pmc/articles/PMC4596548/

Hecht, S.S. "Inhibition of Carcinogenesis by Isothiocyanates." *Drug Metabolism Reviews*, 2000, 32(3–4), 395–411. Accessed Sept. 5, 2019. https://www.ncbi.nlm.nih.gov/pubmed/11139137

Jiang, Y., et al. "Cruciferous Vegetable Intake Is Inversely Correlated with Circulating Levels of Proinflammatory Markers in Women." *Journal of the Academy of Nutrition and*

Dietetics, May 2014, 114(5), 700–708. Accessed Sept. 6, 2019. https://www.ncbi.nlm.nih.gov/pubmed/24630682

Johnson, I.T. "Glucosinolates: Bioavailability and Importance to Health." *International Journal of Vitamin and Nutrition Research*, Jan. 2002, 72(1), 26–31. Accessed Sept. 5, 2019. https://www.ncbi.nlm.nih.gov/pubmed/11887749

Keck, A.S.; and Finley, J.W. "Cruciferous Vegetables: Cancer Protective Mechanisms of Glucosinolate Hydrolysis Products and Selenium." *Integrative Cancer Therapies*, Mar. 2004, 3(1), 5–12. Accessed Sept. 6, 2019. https://www.ncbi.nlm.nih.gov/pubmed/15035868

Oppenheimer, Todd. "The Vegetable Detective." *Craftsmanship*, summer 2015. Accessed Sept. 6, 2019. https://craftsmanship.net/the-vegetable-detective/

Orem, William. "The First Broccoli." Moment of Science, Indiana Public Media, Dec. 29, 2016. Accessed Sept. 6, 2019. https://indianapublicmedia.org/amomentofscience/the-first-broccoli/

Parr, Broderick; Bond, Jennifer K.; and Minor, Travis. "Vegetables and Pulses Outlook: Production Declines and Widening Trade Gap Hinder Per Capita Availability." U.S. Department of Agriculture, May 6, 2019. Accessed Sept. 4, 2019. https://www.ers.usda.gov/webdocs/publications/93033/vgs-362.pdf?v=1958.8

Shahbandeh, M. "Global Production of Vegetables in 2017, by Type (in Million Metric Tons)." Statista, Jan. 28, 2019. Accessed Sept. 4, 2019. https://www.statista.com/statistics/264065/global-production-of-vegetables-by-type/

"Toxicological Review of Thallium and Compounds, CAS No. 7440–28–0." U.S. Environmental Protection Agency, Sept. 2009. Accessed Sept. 6, 2019. https://cfpub.epa.gov/ncea/iris/iris_documents/documents/toxreviews/1012tr.pdf

"US Production of Fresh Vegetables Decreased in 2018." *Vegetable Growers News*, May 22, 2019. Accessed Sept. 4, 2019. https://vegetablegrowersnews.com/news/u-s-production-of-fresh-vegetables-decreased-in-2018/

Villarreal-Garcia, Daniel; and Jacobo-Velazquez, Daniel. "Glucosinolates from Broccoli: Nutraceutical Properties and Their Purification." *Journal of Nutraceuticals and Food Science*, Mar. 10, 2016. Accessed Sept. 6, 2019. http://nutraceuticals.imedpub.com/glucosinolates-from-broccoli-nutraceutical-properties-and-their-purification.php?aid=8986

Dairy Products

WHAT ARE THEY?

Dairy products are foods produced using the milk of mammals. In the United States, these are primarily made from the milk of cows, goats, and sheep, but around the world they may contain milk from water buffaloes, reindeer, horses, camels, donkeys, and a number of others. Milk, cream, cheese, sour cream, cottage cheese, yogurt, ice cream, and butter are some of the most familiar examples of dairy products.

CURRENT CONSUMPTION STATISTICS AND TRENDS

Americans consumed roughly 653 pounds of dairy products per person in 2019, according to the U.S. Department of Agriculture (USDA) Economic Research Service. This includes 141 pounds of milk and other "fluid products" like buttermilk and eggnog, 40.4 pounds of cheeses, 22.4 pounds of ice cream and other frozen milk products, 13.4 pounds of yogurt, and 6.2 pounds of butter. It also encompasses thousands of products that contain dairy ingredients like whey protein, nonfat dry milk, milk protein isolate, sodium caseinate, and milk solids, from baked goods to processed meats.

Annual consumption of dairy products trended upward throughout the 2010s, from 605 pounds per person in 2010 to 646 pounds in 2016, with a slight dip in 2013 as the increase in obesity-related diseases around the world made weight-conscious consumers shy away from full-fat dairy products like butter, cheese, and ice cream. With the increase in dairy soft drinks and single-serving milk products; new dairy snacks like single-serving cottage cheese, cups of Icelandic yogurt, and individually wrapped cheddar squares; varietal products like kefir and kombucha; and more low-fat, nonfat, and protein-fortified choices than ever before, dairy has held onto its market share even as plant-based milk and related products grow their consumer base.

NUTRITIONAL INFORMATION

Dairy products are rich sources of protein and essential amino acids, important nutrients in building and retaining muscle mass. Protein produces a satiated effect, helping people who are dieting feel full longer and crave fewer high-calorie, energy-producing sweets.

These products serve as the body's primary source of calcium, which is required for strong bones and teeth, as well as the vitamin D the body needs to maintain calcium and phosphorus levels. Consumption of dairy products helps the body guard against osteoporosis. Milk and other dairy products are particularly important to children's diets, as they help with bone formation and growth and provide the strength required for muscle growth and development.

Vitamin D, with which many dairy products are fortified, plays a key role in lowering blood pressure, making it a crucial nutrient for heart health. Potassium, vitamin A, riboflavin, vitamin B_{12}, zinc, choline, magnesium, and selenium are all found in dairy products, and all play roles in the body's overall functioning.

HISTORY

Virtually every human child receives milk in one form or another within moments of being born, making it the most basic and prevalent food in human history. The transition away from the mother's breast and to "artificial feeding," using bottles to give babies milk from other mammals, began in earnest at the end of the seventeenth century, according to Mark Kurlansky, author of the book *Milk! A 10,000 Year Food Fracas*. The practice became controversial almost instantly, especially as the public had no understanding of the dangers of spoiled milk—which began to grow bacteria within minutes of leaving the animal. In a world before refrigeration or even the existence of iceboxes, milk became dangerous before it could be consumed or turned into butter or cheese.

In cities in the nineteenth century, landowning residents kept their own cows to provide milk to their families, but as the demand grew, the first large dairy operations began to appear. Stables filled with cows sprang up next door to breweries, where the mash left over from beermaking became feed for many head of cattle. The resulting milk, however, did not have the richness and robust color and texture of the milk to which people had become accustomed, giving rise to "blue milk," a watery substance lacking in fat. "Producers added annatto to improve its color and chalk to give it body," Kurlansky wrote. "They also added water to increase the amount of milk they could sell, and covered up the dilution by adding more chalk."

When widespread cholera in New York City in the 1840s became a death sentence for as many as half the babies in Manhattan, activist Robert Milham Hartley believed that dairies might be playing a role in the spread of disease. He had seen hundreds of dairy stables where cows were kept in miserably unsanitary conditions, were fed "slush" grain devoid of nutrition, and were forced to produce milk even when they were sick and dying. Hartley saw the possibility that the doctored milk—which he dubbed "swill milk"—could have a hand in causing so many babies and children to die in New York, Boston, Philadelphia, and Cincinnati, so he wrote a book in 1842, *An Historical, Scientific, and Practical Essay on Milk, as an Article of Human Sustenance: With a Consideration of the Effects Consequent Upon the Present Unnatural Methods of Producing It for the Supply of Large Cities*, to alert the public to this connection. Another fifteen years would pass, however, before an official report by the Common Council of Brooklyn revealed what Hartley had suspected: Malnourishment and mistreatment of cows too horrific to share here did not provide the nutrition that babies and children needed—in fact, it could well contain diseases that could be passed through the milk to humans. Children by the thousands died of malnutrition, tuberculosis, and other illnesses, while dairy owners made large amounts of money.

In 1862, scientist Louis Pasteur at the University at Lille in France discovered that beverages including beer, wine, and milk became spoiled because of the growth of microorganisms in the liquid. He determined that heating these beverages to a temperature between 60°C and 100°C (140–212°F) killed these bacteria, germs, and mold, making the drinks safe for human consumption. This became the process of pasteurization, but it did not find practical use until German scientist Robert Koch, studying anatomy at the University of Göttingen, discovered that tuberculosis was spread to children through the milk delivered to them by dairies. The dairy industry quickly moved to embrace Koch's work, using the pasteurization process to render the milk safe. Koch went on to develop a way to test cows for tuberculosis; huge numbers of infected cows were removed from dairies, essentially ending the spread of the disease through milk.

A single process did not solve everything that was wrong with milk production, however. Dairies sent delivery people out into neighborhoods on foot with a yoke across their shoulders, on which hung two large, open buckets of milk straight from the cows. All manner of trash could fall into these buckets as they moved from place to place, and did—leaves, twigs, dirt, and so on might be carried in the ladle that delivered milk from the pail to the consumer. Consumers had the option of coming to the dairies and receiving their milk more directly, but this also involved ladling milk out of open buckets. Not until the 1894 invention of the sealed, glass milk bottle by Dr. Henry G. Thatcher of Potsdam, New York, did the industry begin to move toward a more sanitary way of dispensing milk to local consumers.

While scientists and the dairy industry sorted out the issues of milk sanitation and safety, inventor Gail Borden determined a way to condense milk in a vacuum pan so that it could be canned, preserved, and carried great distances without refrigeration. His creation of sweetened condensed milk in cans quickly found customers when it was introduced in 1856, and in 1861, it became an immediate hit with the Union Army as the Civil War began.

Cheese became part of people's daily diet before written recordkeeping began, perhaps some eight thousand years ago when some Mediterranean shepherd must have used a sheep's stomach to carry and store milk. Rennet, an enzyme that occurs naturally in the animal's stomach, would have curdled the milk and turned it into a basic form of cheese. Millennia later, in 4000 BC, Sumerian documents show people eating what could only be cheese, and remnants of some form of cheese have turned up in Egyptian pottery dating back to 2300 BC. Romans developed a process for mass production, learning to culture this substance, age it, give it color and a wide variety of flavors, wrap it in rind, and do many of the other things that dairies do today to create their signature cheeses.

Yogurt, created by fermenting milk using bacteria known as yogurt cultures, is also one of civilization's oldest human-made foods. It gained popularity in Europe and North America in the early 1900s when Russian biologist Ilya Mechnikov, working at the Institut Pasteur in Paris, France, suggested that this staple food of Bulgaria might have something to do with the remarkable longevity of the people there. He took the initiative to spread the word about yogurt throughout Europe, and in 1919, Isaac Carasso developed an industrial process for making yogurt at his business in Barcelona, Spain. He called the business Danone, which later became Dannon as it expanded into the United States. Armenian immigrants Sarkis and Rose Colombosian, living in Andover, Massachusetts, opened their own production facility and called it Colombo and Sons. They delivered their yogurt to homes throughout New England, but it was not until the 1950s that it received national attention as a health food. Looking for a way to expand its popularity to those who found it too sour, the Colombosians added "fruit on the bottom," making yogurt more appetizing to the Western palate and turning it into a confection as well as a healthy option.

THE CONTROVERSY

A great deal of research has explored the question of whether dairy products are good or bad for the human body, with widely differing results.

Some critics begin their argument against dairy with the declaration that consuming milk as an adult is unnatural and unnecessary for good health. Humans are the only animal that consumes the milk of other animals, and we did not do so before agriculture made it possible for us to collect the milk of cattle and other beasts. Only babies should drink milk, critics say, and only from their own mother's breasts.

This theory is borne out by the fact that 75 percent of the world's human population is lactose intolerant, unable to digest milk's most central carbohydrate. This point of view seems logical on its surface, but regional populations in North America, Europe, and Australia seem to have adapted to thousands of years of dairy products in their diets and are well able to digest lactose. In addition, lactose-intolerant people can digest yogurt, which contains probiotic enzymes, as well as aged cheeses that contain no lactose, and some high-fat products like butter.

Not all milk and other dairy products are equal, according to a study that breaks down their composition. In 2008, Helena Lindmark Månsson determined that milk "continuously undergoes changes depending on e.g. breeding, feeding strategies, management of the cow, lactation stage and season." Other studies discovered that cows feeding on green grass produce milk with more omega-3 fatty acids and vitamin K_2 than cows fed on hay and other feed crops. As omega-3 fatty acids help protect against cardiovascular disease and K_2 supports bone health, choosing dairy products from grass-fed cows may be a healthier option than from cows fed on grain.

However, low-fat and nonfat dairy products lose these nutrients—and to maintain the same creamy consistency and flavor as full-fat milk products, producers often add significant amounts of sugar. This essentially negates the benefits that these products provide.

The question of dietary calcium and its role in bone health has been hotly contested over the last several decades. A case control study in Australia, published in 1994, suggested that people who drink milk in their twenties actually increase their risk of hip fracture after age sixty-five. Even the researchers seemed skeptical of their own results, however, as they noted in their report: "Some of the results of this study were unanticipated and may be due to chance or bias. If confirmed by other studies, these results would challenge some current approaches to hip fracture prevention."

A study published in 1997 asked more than 77,000 women to fill out questionnaires in 1980, 1984, and 1986 about their daily dietary intake, as well as about fractures of the thighbone and wrist. The study determined that drinking two or more glasses of milk per day had no more effect on whether these women had a fracture than if they drank one glass or less of milk per week. This was an observational study, however, not one in which milk consumption was actually tested against a control group that did not drink milk, so fractures cannot be considered solely the cause-and-effect results of drinking or not drinking milk.

A string of studies throughout the 1990s produced the opposite result, showing significantly positive effects of drinking milk on bone density in prepubescent girls and both premenopausal and postmenopausal women, while a 2013 study of 3,301 postmenopausal women referred for DEXA bone density screening found that women who reported the lowest dairy intake had the highest incidence of osteoporosis.

In 2016, a paper published in the French journal *Revue du Rhumatisme* completed a literature review of all the studies to date. The team concluded that the studies that asked participants to recall their dietary habits over long periods of time or, in the Australian study's case, as much as fifty years after the fact, could not be seen as valid. "Reliable dietary intake data must be collected over prolonged periods, often long before the occurrence of a fracture, and defective recall may therefore introduce a major yet often unrecognized bias, particularly in populations where calcium deficiency is uncommon," they wrote. "To date, there is no conclusive evidence that we should modify our currently high level of consumption of cow's milk."

What about dairy fat and its effect on obesity and diabetes? Many dairy products contain saturated fat. Studies have shown that the saturated fat in butter is more likely to produce LDL cholesterol in the body than the saturated fat in cheese. A meta-analysis of randomized controlled trials, published in *Nutrition Review* in 2015, showed that butter caused larger concentrations of LDL cholesterol than cheese did.

However, an extensive integration of data from 16 studies, published in the *European Journal of Nutrition* in 2013, determined that consumption of high-fat dairy products actually reduced the risk of obesity and heart disease. "Studies examining the relationship between high-fat dairy consumption and metabolic health reported either an inverse or no association," the authors said. "Studies investigating the connection between high-fat dairy intake and diabetes or cardiovascular disease incidence were inconsistent."

Science struggles with the question of whether or not dairy products are linked to heart disease. Studies work in one of two directions: examining subjects who have already had a heart attack or stroke, working backwards to determine their consumption of dairy products; or attempting to predict a population's risk of heart attack based on how much dairy they eat and drink. Studies also must control for additional risk factors that are known to lead to heart attacks and stroke, including other dietary choices, smoking, and alcohol and drug use.

A study in 2007 looked at dairy fat intake to see if it increased the risk of heart disease, using data from 32,826 subjects in the Nurses' Health Study. Researchers used data from the 166 subjects who actually developed heart disease between the study's launch in 1989 and additional testing in 1996, matching them with 327 control subjects. The team looked for biomarkers of dairy fat intake in the blood of the subjects who had developed heart disease and found high concentrations of these biomarkers. Their conclusion: The biomarkers indicated that "a high intake of dairy fat is associated with a greater risk of [ischemic heart disease]."

An association is not necessarily a causal relationship, however. Other studies have examined the link between drinking milk and heart disease and found the cause-and-effect relationship to be tenuous. A 2004 literature review of cohort studies that featured an estimate of milk and other dairy consumption and vascular disease "provided no convincing evidence that milk is harmful. . . . The studies, taken together, suggest that milk drinking may be associated with a small but worthwhile reduction in heart disease and stroke risk."

A 2010 study involving nearly 4,000 subjects in Costa Rica tested the theory that conjugated linoleic acid (CLA), produced in grass-fed cows' digestive and rumination process, "might offset the adverse effect of the saturated fat content of dairy products." Indeed, the subjects who drank this milk had a lower incidence of heart attacks than those who did not.

Many other meta-analyses of other studies, biomarker studies, and more have attempted to examine specific saturated fats found in dairy products and their effect on heart disease and stroke, but for the most part, their results have been speculative. In short, high-fat dairy products may actually be better for metabolic health than their low-fat and fat-free counterparts—or, as several studies indicate, they may have no effect on heart disease, diabetes, and obesity at all.

None of this has changed the American Heart Association's recommendations on dairy products for heart health, however. The AHA continues to advise no more than two to three servings of fat-free or low-fat dairy products daily for the adult diet and four servings for teenagers and older adults.

FURTHER READINGS

Cumming, R.G.; and Klineberg, R.J. "Case-Control Study of Risk Factors for Hip Fractures in the Elderly." *American Journal of Epidemiology*, Mar. 1, 1994, 139(5), 493–503. Accessed Jan. 19, 2020. https://www.ncbi.nlm.nih.gov/pubmed/8154473

"Dairy Products: Per Capita Consumption, United States (Annual)." Dairy Data, U.S. Department of Agriculture Economic Research Service, Sept. 4, 2020. Accessed Apr.13, 2021. https://www.ers.usda.gov/data-products/dairy-data/

de Goede, J.; Geleijnse, J.M.; Ding, E.L.; and Soedamah-Muthu, S.S. "Effect of Cheese Consumption on Blood Lipids: A Systematic Review and Meta-analysis of Randomized Controlled Trials." *Nutrition Reviews*, 2015, 73(5), 259–275. https://academic.oup.com/nutritionreviews/article/73/5/259/186239

de Vrese, M., et al. "Probiotics—Compensation for Lactase Insufficiency." *American Journal of Clinical Nutrition*, Feb. 2001, 72(2 supplemental), 421S–429S. Accessed Jan. 19, 2020. https://www.ncbi.nlm.nih.gov/pubmed/11157352

Elwood, P.C., et al. "Milk Drinking, Ischaemic Heart Disease and Ischaemic Stroke II. Evidence from Cohort Studies." *European Journal of Clinical Nutrition*, Apr. 24, 2004, 58, 718–724. Accessed Jan. 20, 2020. https://www.nature.com/articles/1601869

Fardellone, Patrice, et al. "Osteoporosis: Is Milk a Kindness or a Curse?" *Revue du Rhumatisme*, Oct. 2016, 83(5), 334–340. Accessed Jan. 19, 2020. https://www.sciencedirect.com/science/article/pii/S1297319X16301178?via%3Dihub

Feskanich, D., et al. "Milk, Dietary Calcium, and Bone Fractures in Women: A 12-Year Prospective Study." *American Journal of Public Health*, June 1997, 87(6), 992–997. Accessed Jan. 19, 2020. https://www.ncbi.nlm.nih.gov/pubmed/9224182

Gunnars, Kris. "Milk and Osteoporosis—Is Dairy Really Good for Your Bones?" Healthline, Apr. 20, 2018. Accessed Jan. 19, 2020. https://www.healthline.com/nutrition/is-dairy-good-for-your-bones#section1

Gunnars, Kris. "Is Dairy Bad for You, or Good? The Milky, Cheesy Truth." Healthline, Nov. 15, 2018. Accessed Jan. 19, 2020. https://www.healthline.com/nutrition/is-dairy-bad-or-good

Hebeisen, D.F., et al. "Increased Concentrations of Omega-3 Fatty Acids in Milk and Platelet Rich Plasma of Grass-Fed Cows." *International Journal of Vitamin and Nutrition Research*, 1993, 63(3), 229–233. Accessed Jan. 19, 2020. https://www.ncbi.nlm.nih.gov/pubmed/7905466

Kratz, Mario, et al. "The Relationship Between High-Fat Dairy Consumption and Obesity, Cardiovascular, and Metabolic Disease." *European Journal of Nutrition*, Feb. 2013, 52(1), 1–24. Accessed Jan. 19, 2020. https://link.springer.com/article/10.1007%2Fs00394-012-0418-1

Kurlansky, Mark. *Milk! A 10,000 Year Food Fracas*. New York: Bloomsbury Publishing, 2019.

Månsson, Helena Lindmark. "Fatty Acids in Bovine Milk Fat." *Food & Nutrition Research*, 2008, 52(10). Accessed Jan. 19, 2020. https://www.ncbi.nlm.nih.gov/pmc/articles/PMC2596709/

"Nutrients and Health Benefits." ChooseMyPlate, U.S. Department of Agriculture. Accessed Jan. 18, 2020. https://www.choosemyplate.gov/eathealthy/dairy/dairy-nutrients-health

Smit, L.A.; Baylin, A.; and Campos, H. "Conjugated Linoleic Acid in Adipose Tissues and Risk of Myocardial Infarction." *American Journal of Clinical Nutrition*, July 2010, 92(1), 34–40. Accessed Jan. 20, 2020. https://www.ncbi.nlm.nih.gov/pubmed/20463040

Soerensen, K.V.; Thorning, T.K.; Astrup, A.; Kristensen, M.; and Lorenzen, J.K. "Effect of Dairy Calcium from Cheese and Milk on Fecal Fat Excretion, Blood Lipids, and Appetite in Young Men." *American Journal of Clinical Nutrition*, 2014, 95(5), 984–991. https://academic.oup.com/ajcn/article/99/5/984/4577518

Sun, Q.; Ma, J.; Campos, H.; and Hu, F.B. "Plasma and Erythrocyte Biomarkers of Dairy Fat Intake and Risk of Ischemic Heart Disease." *American Journal of Clinical Nutrition*, Oct. 2007, 86(4), 929–937. Accessed Jan. 20, 2020. https://www.ncbi.nlm.nih.gov/pubmed/17921367

Tholstrup, T.; Hoy, C.E.; Andersen, L.N.; Christensen, R.D.; and Sandstrom, B. "Does Fat in Milk, Butter and Cheese Affect Blood Lipids and Cholesterol Differently?" *Journal of the American College of Nutrition*, 2004, 23(2), 169–176. https://www.tandfonline.com/doi/abs/10.1080/07315724.2004.10719358

Thorning, Tanja Kongerslev, et al. "Milk and Dairy Products: Good or Bad for Human Health? An Assessment of the Totality of Scientific Evidence." *Food & Nutrition Research*, 2016, 60(10). Accessed Jan. 18, 2020. https://www.ncbi.nlm.nih.gov/pmc/articles/PMC5122229/

Varenna, M., et al. "The Association Between Osteoporosis and Hypertension: The Role of a Low Dairy Intake." *Calcified Tissue International*, July 2013, 93(1), 86–92. Accessed Jan. 19, 2020. https://www.ncbi.nlm.nih.gov/pubmed/23652773

Eggs

WHAT ARE THEY?

The reproduction method for birds, reptiles, amphibians, insects, arachnids, crustaceans, fish, mollusks, and some mammals, eggs have served as food for human beings for thousands of years, since well before recorded history. Nearly all eggs available to U.S. consumers come from chickens, though eggs from other birds are sometimes offered as delicacies. Other cultures may have access to eggs from gulls, guineafowl, ostriches, pheasants, and other birds. Fish eggs (roe or caviar) can be found in many grocery stores and specialty shops. This book focuses on chicken eggs.

CURRENT CONSUMPTION STATISTICS AND TRENDS

United Egg Producers (UEP) reports that 265 million cases of eggs (with thirty dozen eggs per case, for a total of 95.4 billion eggs) were produced in 2018, with 157.6 million cases sold in retail stores and another 90.1 million cases sold to food manufacturers and processors. Another 19.6 million cases went to food service companies. In the United States, people consume roughly 279 eggs per year, including eggs as ingredients in packaged products. This figure has climbed significantly since 2000, in part because the productivity of laying hens has increased through "improved health and disease prevention, nutrition, genetics, and flock management," according to UEP. The removal of cholesterol limits in the 2015–2020 *Dietary Guidelines for Americans* returned eggs to kitchens across the United States, increasing demand from 256.3 per capita in 2015 to 279 in 2019.

NUTRITIONAL INFORMATION

One large chicken egg contains 6 g of protein, as well as significant amounts of riboflavin, vitamin A, niacin, vitamin B_{12}, biotin, vitamin D, iron, pantothenic acid, phosphorus, iodine, zinc, selenium, choline, and antioxidants lutein and zeaxanthin, which have health benefits for vision. It also contains cholesterol and 1.5 g of saturated fat.

HISTORY

Eggs long predated humans, and the date on which they became a human food source cannot possibly be known, but records from ancient Egypt and China both make note of domesticated birds laying eggs for human consumption as far back as 1400 BC. Europe adopted the practice as early as 600 BC, while Christopher Columbus brought chickens on his second voyage to the New World in 1493.

Before the twentieth century, most families either kept their own chickens or purchased eggs directly from private farmers. This began to change in the 1920s, as farmers saw profit in selling eggs and began to increase their own flocks to provide eggs for their neighborhoods or at farmers' markets in nearby towns and cities. Large numbers of chickens living in close quarters began to pose issues for farmers, however, as hens naturally established a pecking order—hence the name—and the larger and stronger birds gobbled up most of the food farmers provided. Chicken hatcheries became early adopters of selective breeding, choosing the healthiest hens to produce chicks that would become the next generation of layers.

Chickens lived outdoors for the most part, a situation that resulted in losses to predators and weather. Keeping chicken pens clean and protecting the birds from parasites also became significant problems for farmers, so when research on indoor hen houses demonstrated that the cost of the houses would be recouped in dramatically reduced losses of birds, farmers moved to these specialized quarters in droves. "Indoor houses . . . helped to prevent parasite infestations and reduce the spread of diseases from outside carriers, including rodents and even humans," the American Egg Board explains in a concise history of commercial egg production. "Instead of hens eating whatever they found outside, feed could be better controlled indoors, too." By the 1940s, most hen houses supplied wire housing for each bird, moving them off the floor and making it easier for each hen to get the nutrition she needed, rather than battling other hens for her share of the feed. Farmers found it easier to keep the houses clean with the birds living in cages. Healthier hens laid more eggs, so the houses soon required conveyor belts to collect the eggs and move them to the egg washing system. Egg producing facilities grew exponentially under these conditions, until they reached the size they are today, with as many as one million birds in a single flock and more than 280 million hens across the United States.

Meanwhile, nutrition scientists had begun to explore the link between blood lipids and heart health and had discovered a causal relationship between high cholesterol and heart disease. Most common knowledge in the scientific community in the first half of the twentieth century indicated that rising cholesterol levels were simply a fact of aging, so the possibility that food choices and eating patterns might cause high cholesterol had not been considered by most researchers. This changed in 1955 when Ancel Keys at the University of Minnesota suggested:

> There is an important relationship between the concentration of certain lipid fractions in the blood and the development of atherosclerosis and the coronary heart disease it produces. The outstanding characteristic of atherosclerosis is the presence of lipid deposits, mainly cholesterol, in the walls of the arteries. And both in man and animals the most obvious factor that affects the blood lipids is the diet.

Studies began to explore this connection, and as the research produced a correlation between cholesterol and heart disease, the American Heart Association took the bold step in 1968 of recommending that people consume no more than 300 mg of cholesterol in their diet per day and no more than three whole eggs per week.

In 1973, researchers began the landmark Coronary Primary Prevention Trial (CPPT), a sixteen-year randomized double-blind trial that tested the effectiveness of reducing the risk of CHD by lowering cholesterol. The study showed that lowering LDL levels in men could reduce the incidence of mortality from heart disease, providing "strong evidence for a causal role for these lipids in the pathogenesis of CHD." This opened the door to the development of cholesterol-lowering pharmaceuticals, but it would take decades before the egg found its way back to American dining tables.

THE CONTROVERSY

Once the American Heart Association labeled the egg yolk as the highest cholesterol food in most people's diets in 1968, the egg industry began to see a marked decline in sales. After the CPPT published findings that a pharmaceutical solution to high cholesterol could help guard against heart disease, the egg had a chance for a comeback—but on March 26, 1984, *Time* magazine published a cover photo of a dinner-plate face, with a frowning bacon-strip mouth and two fried eggs for eyes. The headline: "Cholesterol: And Now for The Bad News."

The industry had several options: It could accept its fate and begin to downsize to keep pace with the dwindling demand or it could fight back—but any effort to discredit the cholesterol findings could be seen as putting its own profits before the health of its customers. If it chose to fund its own research, however, the results would be seen as nothing more than a special interest group trying to rationalize or even negate highly credible and legitimate science—science, in fact, that had resulted in a 1985 Nobel Prize for its lead researchers.

As bad press for the egg mounted—with the Select Committee on Nutrition, the National Cholesterol Education Program of the Heart, Lung, and Blood Institute, and a wide range of nongovernment organizations piling on—the egg industry responded. First, it produced an egg substitute product: Egg Beaters, which contains egg whites and added thickeners (see guar gum and xanthan gum in this book), but leaves out the high-cholesterol egg yolk. Egg Beaters was introduced in 1972 and continues to be a popular product with people working to lower their LDL levels. Its success soon generated a number of similar products, including many flavored varieties and egg whites in pourable form.

In 1984, the egg industry created the Egg Nutrition Center (ENC). The ENC operated separately from the commercial side of egg production, forming its own advisory panel of university-based scientists to put together a long-range research plan.

Rather than attempt to disprove the many dietary guidelines that limited eggs, the ENC's researchers began by focusing on eggs as a low-cost, nutrient-rich protein source, as well as on their role in aiding people in maintaining a healthy weight. Results of studies emphasized the role of eggs in helping elderly consumers preserve muscle tissue mass and the importance of antioxidants lutein and zeaxanthin, supplied by eggs in abundance, in combatting cataracts and macular degeneration. Research determined that eggs contain choline, an essential nutrient for fetal and neonatal brain development, that is often lacking in pregnant women's diet.

More recently, studies funded by the ENC, as well as by the Centers for Disease Control and Prevention or the National Institutes of Health, began to generate good news for egg producers. A cohort review published in 2007 looked at 9,734 adults aged twenty-five to seventy-four to find a link between egg consumption and cardiovascular disease. Researchers categorized egg consumption into groups: those who ate less than one egg per week, those who ate one to six eggs, and a final group who ate more than six eggs weekly. The report concluded:

> After adjusting for differences in age, gender, race, serum cholesterol level, body mass index, diabetes mellitus, systolic blood pressure, educational status and cigarette smoking, no significant difference was observed between persons who consumed greater than 6 eggs per week compared to those who consume none or less than 1 egg per week in regards to any stroke . . . or coronary artery disease. Consumption of greater than six eggs per week (average of one egg or greater per day) does not increase the risk of stroke and ischemic stroke.

In 2010, Valentine Njike et al. completed a randomized, placebo-controlled crossover trial of forty adults with high cholesterol. The subjects first ate a single "dose" of three hardboiled eggs or a sausage and cheese breakfast sandwich and then tested the function of the endothelium—the lining of blood vessels, a well-known factor in heart disease. Neither high-cholesterol meal had any effect on endothelial function. Next, the subjects ate either a half-cup of cooked Egg Beaters or two eggs daily for six weeks and found that eating eggs had no effect on cholesterol levels. Eating Egg Beaters, however, did indeed lower the subjects' cholesterol.

In 2015, in a randomized, controlled crossover trial of thirty-two adults with diagnosed cardiovascular disease, Katz et al. tested three different breakfast options: a meal with two eggs, a meal with half a cup of cooked Egg Beaters, and a high carbohydrate breakfast with no eggs. The subjects ate the assigned breakfast daily for six weeks and found that eating two eggs daily had no effect on blood pressure, cholesterol, or body weight. "No outcomes differed (P >.05) between eggs and Egg Beaters," the study concluded.

One of the most recent cohort studies took place in China, recruiting more than 500,000 adults from ten different regions and following them for nine years. Researchers surveyed the health and eating habits of this enormous base of participants and found that "daily egg consumption was associated with a lower risk of [cardiovascular disease]. . . . Among Chinese adults, a moderate level of egg consumption (up to <1 egg/day) was significantly associated with lower risk of CVD, largely independent of other risk factors."

The mounting evidence had the desired effect: When the 2015–2020 *Dietary Guidelines for Americans* arrived in 2015, it contained no specific restriction on egg consumption. Eggs are now included in the guidelines as a protein choice. Even the American Heart Association has moved away from its prohibition of eggs: Its guidelines now suggest one egg or two egg whites daily can be part of a heart-healthy diet and more for vegetarians who may be consuming eggs as their only source of protein.

FURTHER READINGS

American Heart Association News. "Are Eggs Good For You Or Not?" American Heart Association, Aug. 16, 2018. Accessed Jan. 21, 2020. https://www.heart.org/en/news/2018/08/15/are-eggs-good-for-you-or-not

Chenxi, Qin, et al. "Associations of Egg Consumption with Cardiovascular Disease in a Cohort Study of 0.5 Million Chinese Adults." *Heart*, Nov. 2018, 104(21). Accessed Jan. 21, 2020. https://heart.bmj.com/content/104/21/1756

"Cholesterol: And Now for the Bad News." *Time Magazine*, Mar. 26, 1984, cover. Accessed Jan. 20, 2020. http://content.time.com/time/covers/0,16641,19840326,00.html

"Egg Nutrition Facts Labels." Egg Nutrition Center, June 2019. Accessed Jan. 20, 2020. https://www.eggnutritioncenter.org/egg-nutrition-facts-panels/

"Facts and Stats." United Egg Producers, 2019. Accessed Jan. 20, 2020. https://unitedegg.com/facts-stats/

Garbarino, Jeanne. "Cholesterol and Controversy: Past, Present and Future." *Scientific American*, Nov. 15, 2011. Accessed Jan. 20, 2020. https://blogs.scientificamerican.com/guest-blog/cholesterol-confusion-and-why-we-should-rethink-our-approach-to-statin-therapy/

"History of Commercial Egg Production." American Egg Board. Accessed Jan. 20, 2020. https://www.aeb.org/farmers-and-marketers/history-of-egg-production

Katz, David L., et al. "Effects of Egg Ingestion on Endothelial Function in Adults with Coronary Artery Disease: A Randomized, Controlled, Crossover Trial." *American Heart Journal*, Jan. 2015, 169(1), 162–169. Accessed Jan. 21, 2020. https://www.sciencedirect.com/science/article/abs/pii/S0002870314006048

Keys, Ancel, et al. "Effects of Diet on Blood Lipids in Man, Particularly Cholesterol and Lipoproteins." *Clinical Chemistry*, 1(1), 1955, 34–52. Accessed Jan. 20, 2020. http://clinchem.aaccjnls.org/content/clinchem/1/1/34.full.pdf

"Lipid Research Clinics (LRC) Coronary Primary Prevention Trial (CPPT)." National Heart, Lung, and Blood Institute. Accessed Jan. 20, 2020. https://biolincc.nhlbi.nih.gov/studies/lrccppt/

McNamera, Donald J. "The Fifty Year Rehabilitation of the Egg." *Nutrients*, Oct. 2015, 7(10), 8716–8722. Accessed Jan. 20, 2020. https://www.ncbi.nlm.nih.gov/pmc/articles/PMC4632449/

Njike, Valentine, et al. "Daily Egg Consumption in Hyperlipidemic Adults—Effects on Endothelial Function and Cardiovascular Risk." *Nutrition Journal*, 2010, 9(28). Accessed Jan. 21, 2020. https://www.ncbi.nlm.nih.gov/pmc/articles/PMC2904713/?report=reader

Qureshi, Al, et al. "Regular Eff Consumption Does Not Increase the Risk of Stroke and Cardiovascular Diseases." *Medical Science Monitor*, Jan. 2007, 13(1), CR1–CR8. Accessed Jan. 21, 2020. https://www.ncbi.nlm.nih.gov/pubmed/17179903

Shahbandeh, M. "Per Capita Consumption of Eggs in the United States from 2000 to 2019." Statista, Aug. 9, 2019. Accessed Jan. 20, 2020. https://www.statista.com/statistics/183678/per-capita-consumption-of-eggs-in-the-us-since-2000/

"Suggested Servings from Each Food Group." American Heart Association. Accessed Jan. 21, 2020. https://www.heart.org/en/healthy-living/healthy-eating/eat-smart/nutrition-basics/suggested-servings-from-each-food-group

Essential Oils

WHAT ARE THEY?

Essential oils are distillations of the hydrocarbons (terpenes) in plant matter, the molecules that give the plant its scent. They are obtained from the plant through one of a number of distillation methods or through cold-pressing, also known as expression. A few are extracted using alcohol or another solvent. They are called essential oils because the processing extracts their essence, or scent—not because they are somehow essential to life or health.

CURRENT CONSUMPTION STATISTICS AND TRENDS

With hundreds of different products in the essential oils market, sales statistics are divided into market segments—and specific information about them is well guarded behind paywalls at market research firms. The food and beverage market appears to be the fastest growing niche for essential oils, however, with demand growing since 2015 and expected to continue through the 2020s. These oils are sold in the pharmaceuticals, cosmetics, personal care, spa and salon, household cleaning, and food and beverages markets, and growth is expected to reach $9.6 billion by 2022, according to multiple research reports.

NUTRITIONAL INFORMATION

While many claims have been made about the healing properties and other effects of essential oils, they have no nutritional value in terms of calories, vitamins, minerals, protein, carbohydrates, or any other nutrients.

HISTORY

The use of plants for flavoring and seasoning food began long ago, but specific mention of early precursors to essential oils appeared around 1800 BC, when Greek and Roman physicians visited Egypt to study advances in medicine there. Distillation of these plant essences began with Avicenna, an early Persian scientist, who determined a method for doing this sometime after AD 980 AD. The oils that resulted were in common medicinal use well into the nineteenth century. In 1881, Dela Croix was the first to find that essential oil vapors had bactericidal properties, but interest in this research waned as modern pharmaceuticals and their dependable results largely replaced essential oils in the general apothecary.

French fragrance chemist René-Maurice Gattefossé turned his attention to the study of essential oils' therapeutic uses in 1910, when an explosion in his laboratory sprayed burning liquid onto his hands. He ran out to the lawn and rolled on the ground until he extinguished the flames, but when he saw that his hands were infected with gas gangrene, he rinsed them with lavender essence and "stopped the gasification of the tissue," he wrote in his book, *Aromatherapy*, in 1937. Gattefossé took a professional interest in researching essential oils from then on, publishing books and articles on the topic.

Essential oils remained in the *United States Pharmacopeia* until the Food, Drugs and Cosmetics Act was signed into law in 1938, requiring the U.S. FDA to approve every drug before it could be brought to market. While the Bureau of Plant Industry under the U.S. Department of Agriculture conducted a number of studies on plants from which essential oils are distilled throughout the first half of the twentieth century, none of these oils remained on the approved pharmaceuticals list—though it is unclear whether the bureau found them to be ineffective or simply studied the oils for their food flavoring abilities rather than their medicinal properties.

Essential oils saw a rebirth in the latter half of the twentieth century, as multilevel marketing corporations including Young Living and doTerra engaged millions of consumers in using these products as alternatives to prescription medications as well as for aromatherapy and household cleaning. Consumers looking to replace chemicals in their homes with natural solutions embraced essential oils and the many claims these marketing companies made about their effectiveness.

In the late twentieth and early twenty-first centuries, as the demand for organic foods and "clean" foods have reduced the use of artificial ingredients by some manufacturers, essential oils have risen in popularity as additives for processed and packaged foods, both to add flavor and aroma to soft drinks and other foods and as alternatives to synthetic preservatives. The food industry has taken significant interest in essential oils, and many studies in the 2000s and 2010s explored their possible antimicrobial and antioxidative properties to determine their usefulness in food packaging. This research continues and has yielded some promising results.

THE CONTROVERSY

Over the last half-century, essential oils have generated a great deal of conflict between factions who believe that their natural origins make them superior to Western medicine and those who see them as nothing more than the snake oil of old-time peddlers. Multilevel marketing programs that make promises of healing properties through aromatherapy, topical application, and other home uses have placed these products on the same plane with healing crystals, copper bracelets, and psychic readings in the minds of more scientifically minded individuals.

The food industry, however, has spent considerable time and money exploring the possibility that essential oils could replace many synthetic preservatives in processed foods. A PubMed search in late 2020 produced a staggering 21,834 results for papers about studies involving essential oils, a pinnacle reached after a decade of significantly increased interest in the topic. "Consumers' concern regarding possible negative health effects of applying synthetic preservatives to food products, together with the boom of organic culture that promotes the consumption of organic foods (in whose processing synthetic additives are not authorized), have . . . contribute[d] to boost the interest in organic [essential oils'] properties," wrote Juana Fernández-López and Manuel Viuda-Martos in their introduction to the special April 2018 issue of the journal *Foods*, on essential oils in food systems.

As it turns out, these oils may actually have the antimicrobial and antioxidative properties their marketers have claimed for decades, potentially making them effective in extending the shelf life of many foods. For example, in 2018, a study of the properties of an assortment of essential oils harvested in a region of Italy (including rosemary, oregano, salvia, peppermint, garlic, fennel, savory, thyme, and coriander) showed "interesting biological potentiality," according to the team's report, indicating that further laboratory work "could be used to define these essential oils as potential candidates for natural biopreservatives in combination with or in substitution to synthetic chemical ones" (Pellegrini et al.). Another in vitro study examined the antibacterial and antioxidant activity of four varieties of thyme essential oil and found that two of them—*Thymus zygis* and *Thymus capitatus*—showed the highest antibacterial activity, particularly when tested on beef. In 2017, Carmen Ballester-Costa et al. concluded that these two oils "may be used, by the food industry in general and the meat industry in particular, as potential natural or 'green' additives to replace or reduce the use of chemical ones." The next step, they added, would be to determine which essential oil would have the greatest preservative effect on each type of food.

In 2018, Houda Banani et al. tested thyme and savory essential oils' ability to increase the resistance of fruit—in this case, apples—to the gray mold *Botrytis cinerea* and found that the treated apples "showed significantly lower gray mold severity and incidence." The research team determined that the oils prime the apple's own defense response to *B. cinerea*, causing the apple to produce pathogenesis-related gene PR-8, which protects the apple from the mold.

Replacing synthetic preservatives with essential oils is not as simple as it sounds, however. "The first method of application was directly added essential oil to the food matrix, which showed special limitations," posed by "their low water solubility, high volatility, low stability, bioavailability, and strong odor," Fernández-López and Viuda-Martos said. The oils are inherently unstable and "can be degraded easily . . . when they are added to the food matrix. It must be taken into account that most of the food elaboration processes include heat treatment or air and light exposition, all of the factors that increase their degradation."

One solution may be to add the oils to the food packaging rather than to the food itself, incorporating them into edible films and coatings. "The effectiveness of the edible film against microbial growth will depend on the oil's nature and the type of microorganism," the article continued. Research continues into this and a wide range of other possibilities that may lead to essential oils replacing chemical synthetics in food production, especially in the organic food sector.

In addition, food-grade essential oils have long been ingredients in packaged food products. Food-grade oils are required to have nutrition information on their packaging, making them distinctly different from the oils used in aromatherapy; they also may be combined with vegetable glycerine or propylene glycol (an organic compound) to make them easier to use in food preparation. A total of 144 essential oils are GRAS by the FDA and have received approval for use as food flavorings.

The oils available for topical use and aromatherapy use are not appropriate for use in food and should not be ingested, as the distributors usually note in their literature. The FDA provides food manufacturers with specific instructions for the types of essential oils that can be used as food additives and flavorings and how much of each form is safe. Food-grade essential oils can be purchased by consumers for use as flavorings; they are much stronger than the extracts sold in supermarkets and must be used very sparingly to achieve the desired flavor.

FURTHER READINGS

Ballester-Costa, Carmen, et al. "Assessment of Antioxidant and Antibacterial Properties on Meat Homogenates of Essential Oils Obtained from Four Thymus Species Achieved from Organic Growth." *Foods*, Aug. 2017, 6(8). Accessed Jan. 22, 2020. https://www.ncbi.nlm.nih.gov/pmc/articles/PMC5575634/?report=reader

Banani, Houda, et al. "Thyme and Savory Essential Oil Efficacy and Induction of Resistance Against Botrytis cinerea Through Priming of Defense Responses in Apple." *Foods*, Feb. 2018, 7(2). Accessed Jan. 22, 2020. https://www.ncbi.nlm.nih.gov/pmc/articles/PMC5848115/?report=reader

"Essential Oils Market, For Food & Beverages, Pharmaceuticals, Cosmetics & Personal Care Products, Spa And Salon Products, Household Cleaning Products And

Other Applications Is Expected to Reach Over US$ 9.6 Bn by 2022." *Credence Research*, July 2016. Accessed Jan. 21, 2020. https://www.credenceresearch.com/press/global-essential-oils-market

Fernández-López, Juana; and Viuda-Martos, Manuel. "Introduction to the Special Issue: Application of Essential Oils in Food Systems." *Foods*, Apr. 2018, 7(4), 56. Accessed Jan. 21, 2020. https://www.ncbi.nlm.nih.gov/pmc/articles/PMC5920421/

"Food Additive Status List." U.S. Food and Drug Administration, Oct. 24, 2019. Accessed Jan. 21, 2020. https://www.fda.gov/food/food-additives-petitions/food-additive-status-list#ftnE

Minetor, Randi. *Essential Oils and Aromatherapy: An Introductory Guide*. Berkeley, CA: Sonoma Press, 2014.

Pellegrini, Marika, et al. "Characterization of Essential Oils Obtained from Abruzzo Autochthonous Plants: Antioxidant and Antimicrobial Activities Assessment for Food Application." *Foods*, Feb. 2018, 7(2). Accessed Jan. 21, 2020. https://www.ncbi.nlm.nih.gov/pmc/articles/PMC5848123/?report=reader

Peter, K.V., ed. *Handbook of Herbs and Spices*. Elsevier, 2012, p. 18.

Preedy, Victor, ed. *Essential Oils in Food Preservation, Flavor and Safety*. Cambridge, MA: Academic Press, 2016.

Sendra, Esther. "Essential Oils in Foods: From Ancient Times to the 21st Century." *Foods*, June 2016, 5(2). Accessed Jan. 21, 2020. https://www.ncbi.nlm.nih.gov/pmc/articles/PMC5302348/

"Super Strength Candy Oils & Food Grade Essential Oils." LorAnn Oils. Accessed Jan. 22, 2020. https://www.lorannoils.com/food-grade-essential-oils-super-strength-flavors

Tippen, Brenda. "The Real Story of René-Maurice Gattefossé—Essential Oils During the Past Century Part II." Oilwellessentials4health, Feb. 2, 2016. Accessed Jan. 21, 2020. https://oilwellessentials4health.wordpress.com/2016/02/02/the-real-story-of-rene-maurice-gattefosse-essential-oils-during-the-past-century-part-ii/

Tippen, Brenda. "Forgotten: Essential Oils and the US Government's Little Known Role—Essential Oils During the Past Century III." Oilwellessentials4health, Feb. 8, 2016. Accessed Jan. 22, 2020. https://oilwellessentials4health.wordpress.com/2016/02/08/forgotten-essential-oils-and-the-us-governments-little-known-role-essential-oils-during-the-past-century-part-iii/

Wormwood, Valerie Ann. *The Complete Book of Essential Oils and Aromatherapy*. New World Library, Aug. 23, 2012, p. 9.

Farm-Raised Fish and Seafood

WHAT IS IT?

Farm-raised fish and seafood are raised commercially in enclosures in lakes, rivers, or oceans, or in large tanks. Fish and seafood farming is known as aquaculture, and fish raised in this manner are more easily accessible to supermarkets, fish markets, restaurants, and consumers than wild-caught fish—and are usually less expensive. While fish in the wild catch and eat what they find—insects, plankton, invertebrates, small fish, squid, eels, and shrimp, for example—farm-raised fish are fed fortified feed, often in the form of dried pellets, which contain the vitamins, minerals, amino acids, and fats each fish species requires for optimum health and growth.

CURRENT CONSUMPTION STATISTICS AND TRENDS

In the United States, seafood consumption in general has been on a decline since 2006, when it reached a record high of 16.5 pounds per person annually. In 2018, consumption had fallen to 14.9 pounds per person. (For comparison, the U.S. annual per capita consumption of chicken in 2018 was 90.1 pounds and beef was 55.4 pounds.) Of this, about 55 percent of all seafood consumed in 2017 included three types: shrimp, canned tuna, and salmon. Tilapia, Alaskan pollock, pangasius, cod, crab, catfish, and clams make up the rest of the top ten seafood products consumed.

In 2017, 633 million pounds of farm-raised fish and shellfish were produced in the United States. "In the United States, the amount of fish and shellfish harvested from the wild annually is more than ten times greater than the amount produced by domestic aquaculture farms," the Community Seafood Initiative reported on its website in 2020. In 2018, aquaculture was a $1.5 billion industry in the United States, according to the USDA's National Agricultural Statistics Service, with food fish representing $716 million, mollusks (shellfish) $441.8 million, and crustaceans (lobsters and crawfish) $100.4 million. Catfish is the single most popular food fish at 51 percent of sales, while oysters are the top seller in mollusks, accounting for 64 percent of shellfish sales.

NUTRITIONAL INFORMATION

All fish and shellfish contain omega-3 fatty acids, which limit the ability of blood to clot within blood vessels, reducing the likelihood of heart attack or stroke. Omega-3s also play a role in decreasing the risk of depression, ADHD, Alzheimer's disease, other forms of dementia, and diabetes and may reduce inflammation within the body. Fattier fish, including salmon, herring, and mackerel, contain more than 1,500 mg of omega-3s per 3-ounce cooked portion, whether the fish are wild-caught or farmed. Farmed fish may contain slightly higher levels of omega-3s, both because the food they eat may be fortified to produce higher levels and because farm-raised salmon tend to be fattier than wild-caught salmon. As the human body does not make its own omega-3s, fish are an important source of this nutrient.

Fish also contain vitamin D, riboflavin (B_2), calcium, phosphorus, iron, zinc, iodine, magnesium, potassium, and high-quality protein. The American Heart Association recommends eating two to three 3.5-ounce servings of fish every week, especially salmon, mackerel, herring, lake trout, sardines, and albacore tuna.

HISTORY

Aquaculture—the practice of farm-raising fish—may seem like a fairly recent phenomenon, but it actually began thousands of years ago. Historians theorize that it may have started when people discovered that oxbows—deep curves in rivers—trapped fish and other organisms in waterways left behind when floodwaters receded with the seasons and after storms. The same may have been true in tropical areas, where monsoons flooded low-lying areas for part of the year, creating easy fishing until the fields dried out. This ability to contain fish in one place made them fairly effortless to catch and may have led to the practice of actually moving fish to these contained areas to increase the variety of species. Stocking fish in ponds, streams, and moats began in medieval times, when rulers of empires demanded fish year-round as part of their diet; those procuring food for the wealthy and powerful made certain that fish were always available by transferring wild fish to contained waterways and raising them there. Along seashores, fishermen knew of inlets and lagoons that formed natural containers for fish and mollusks and barricaded these to keep the fish inside, allowing them to grow to a size suitable for harvest. All of these were primitive forms of fish farming, using natural resources and turning them to human advantage.

China receives credit as the first cradle of aquaculture, with beginnings between 2000 and 1000 BC. The Chinese bred common carp in captivity as the nation's populations created centers of civilization, forsaking their largely nomadic lifestyle in favor of agriculture. Somewhere around 475 BC, politician-turned-fish-farmer Fan Lai (also spelled Li or Lee) wrote a monograph called "The Chinese Fish Culture Classic," the first written instructions for aquatic husbandry, providing information about raising mass quantities of fish for sale and consumption.

The first records of fish breeding in reservoirs built for this purpose appeared between 321 and 300 BC in the Indian subcontinent. Farming fish was a well-established practice in China by this time, widening from common carp to several other species between AD 600 and 900. Fish farmers collected fry (juvenile fish) of species they wanted to raise along the rivers, transporting them to their reservoirs to grow into maturity.

The rise of Christianity in the Middle Ages pushed Europeans toward fish farming, particularly near monasteries where eating meat was forbidden by faith on many days throughout the year. Along the southern European coastline, fish farmers built rudimentary enclosures in lagoons and ponds where the tides swept in fish and mollusks, keeping them in brackish water for harvesting.

By the thirteenth century, Indian fish farmer Namasollasa wrote his description of the process for fattening fish in reservoirs, and Chinese writers documented their own aquaculture processes in a number of manuscripts. *The Complete Book of Agriculture*, a Chinese publication, was published in 1639 with a substantial section on pond fish culture.

The methods of fish farming made their move toward today's practices in 1741, when German scientist Stephen Ludwig Jacobi built the first fish hatchery—a trout operation in Westphalia. He raised the resulting fish for food, proving that fish could be produced in this manner. By this time, fish producers had moved away from using natural lagoons and the tides or weather to capture whatever fish happened to drift their way and had begun to introduce fry into these impoundments. They also determined what kinds of feed would produce meatier fish and began to control what and how much the fish ate.

Nearly 100 years passed before Jacobi's fish hatchery methods took hold throughout Europe and North America. The effects of the Industrial Revolution depleted much of the world's freshwater fish supply, so hatcheries were engaged to resupply these continents with fish. North American fish farming did not get underway until the nineteenth century, when its emphasis was on stocking wilderness ponds, rivers, and streams for sport fishing. To this end, the U.S. Commission of Fish and Fisheries published *A Manual of Fish Culture* in 1897. Meanwhile, the U.S. fish farmers had very good luck with rainbow trout, which thrived in hatcheries and tanks and soon became a dominant fish in Europe as well.

In the twentieth century, aquaculture expanded quickly with the opening of fish hatcheries to spawn the species most popular for food. A Japanese innovation, the floating cage, made it possible to hold fish captive in a large net attached to the bottom of a natural waterway, with a circular frame floating on top of the water to define the space. European fisheries embraced this new method, bringing rainbow trout into the Norwegian fjords and Atlantic salmon into the ocean waters. Salmon farming boomed in the 1970s and 1980s in Europe, especially in Norway and Scotland, while countries along the Mediterranean Sea farmed salmon, seabass, and seabream. In the 1990s, fisheries began using tanks filled with seawater to farm flatfishes, which need to rest on the bottom of the sea or lake.

Today fish farming is a $1.5 billion industry in the United States. The demand for fish and seafood has pushed the "fed" segment of the industry—fish that do not find all the nutrients they need in the water, and so must be fed by fish farmers—into growth beyond the waters of each state, with some fisheries looking to expand into federal waters (oceans) to keep up with demand.

THE CONTROVERSY

Aquaculture offers a critically important solution to overfishing the world's waterways and oceans, pollution's impact on the seafood supply, and the changes in our rivers, lakes, and oceans driven by climate change. As the planet's population continues to grow, providing an abundant food supply to billions of people is a top priority, and farm-raised fish and seafood can play a leading role in doing so.

In the 2000s and 2010s, as aquaculture became an increasingly larger force in the American food supply, practices were introduced that led to many questions about the safety and advisability of eating farm-raised fish and seafood.

A 2004 study published in *Science* (Hites et al.) analyzed the content of more than two metric tons of farmed and wild salmon and found that the farmed salmon contained "significantly higher" concentrations of organochlorines (chemicals used in manufacturing many products and as pesticides) than wild-caught salmon—especially salmon raised in European waters. "Risk analysis indicates that consumption of farmed Atlantic salmon may pose health risks that detract from the beneficial effects of fish consumption," the study concluded.

The most prevalent of these chemicals were polychlorinated biphenyl (PCBs), as already proved by a 2003 study completed by the Environmental Working Group (EWG). A known carcinogen, PCBs were banned in the United States in 1979, but they remain in the environment for decades. "EWG analysis of state-of-the-art fish consumption data derived from 20,000 adults from 1990 through 2002 shows that roughly 800,000 U.S. adults are 100 times over their lifetime allowable cancer risk by eating this contaminated salmon," the report said. "Farmed salmon are fattened with ground fishmeal and fish oils that are high in PCBs. As a result, salmon farming operations that produce inexpensive fish unnaturally concentrate PCBs and have a higher fat content."

The fishmeal in salmon's food back in 2003 and 2004 came from small "feeder" fish harvested from the ocean, where these fish encountered PCBs in their own natural food supply. Since then, farmed salmon feed has changed significantly with the goal of eliminating as much of the PCBs and other contaminants as possible. Levels of fishmeal and fish oil in salmon food pellets have diminished significantly, from 52 percent in 2000 to 26 percent in 2013.

All of this being said, there has been no study of United States fisheries to date that refreshes the data about farmed fish and PCBs. The original study's methodology was particularly costly, making it difficult to obtain the necessary funding to duplicate it, even though the results could be invaluable to fish farms and consumers alike. The question of which governing body should conduct the study also comes into play, as the fish farming industry falls under no less than six federal agencies in the United States alone.

One study conducted by a team of Polish researchers in 2020, published in the *Journal of Veterinary Research*, tested fish raised in Polish and Vietnamese farms for PCBs and dioxins, another chemical with the potential to harm humans. The testing resulted in chemical levels that were "low in relation to maximum limits," but the report noted that two portions of fish per week could still result in levels as much as 866 percent above "tolerable weekly intake (TWI)" for children, and 286 percent above TWI for adults (Mikolajczyk et al., 2020). How this may compare to farmed fish in the United States, however, is unknown.

Consumers with a fondness for salmon can find the most recent dietary guidelines for eating farmed fish on the Mayo Clinic and Seafood Health Facts websites.

Another leading concern involves the levels of antibiotics used to keep these fish healthy. In some fisheries, the fish are raised in underwater pens that keep the fish at close quarters with one another, making the spread of illness a virtual certainty if fishery management does not take steps to prevent it. Such proximity and restricted movement also causes a buildup of waste, which contributes to the spread of disease.

A short list of antibiotics to guard against infection or illness is approved for use with finfish by the U.S. FDA and regulators in countries around the world. (Shellfish do not require antibiotics.) The FDA requires, however, that the fish producers stop administering antibiotics 30–180 days before the fish are sold. This interval assures that the drugs have left the fish's systems or at least are well below the level approved by the FDA as safe before they are harvested for food.

Even with this rule in place, a very limited study conducted by Arizona State University's Biodesign Institute in 2014 found trace amounts of five antibiotics in samples of fish purchased at grocery stores in Arizona and California. The researchers purchased just twenty-seven samples originating in eleven countries and tested them for forty-seven different antibiotics, turning up five: oxytetracycline in farmed tilapia, salmon, and trout; 4-epioxytetracycline in farmed salmon; sulfadimethoxine in farmed shrimp; ormetoprim in farmed salmon; and virginiamycin in farmed salmon that had been labeled antibiotic-free. "All seafood analyzed was found to be in compliance with U.S. FDA regulations," an article about the study in *Aquaculture North America* said. "However, the authors note that sub-regulatory antibiotic levels can promote resistance development in microbes. . . . Because many antibiotics (such as amoxicillin and ampicillin) used in aquaculture are also used in human medicine, proper monitoring of antibiotic residences in seafood is critical, the authors point out." (Neither amoxicillin nor ampicillin was found in the samples.)

The fact that antibiotics are used in farm-raised fish was hardly news, as 80 percent of all antibiotics used in the United States alone are used on livestock, according to the National Consumers League. The study raised the visibility of an already sensitive issue, however. Fish raised in large net pens in major waterways can interact with wild fish, which can swallow fish food pellets and come into contact with fish waste that contains antibiotics. The fish waste also transmits these drugs to surrounding plants and invertebrates in the water, impacting other species.

Does any of this affect human beings eating farm-raised fish? Antibiotics in food may be leading to the evolution of drug-resistant bacteria, which could make future diseases harder to treat. This overexposure can also make current antibiotics less effective.

Setting up wild-caught fish as a healthier option, however, may not actually be valid reasoning. With the world's oceans stressed by overfishing and overharvesting of seafood, plastics pollution, and rising waters from melting polar ice caps and permafrost, wild-caught saltwater fish may not be a sustainable option.

Many states, especially those without oceanfront, have regulations that make fish farming environmentally friendly and less vulnerable to the diseases spread by fish in close quarters. Fish raised in raceways—manmade outdoor systems with fast-flowing water that removes waste—or in indoor recirculating ponds have much less exposure to bacteria than do fish in net enclosures in lakes. Aquaponics facilities are indoor ponds in which plants grow along with the fish, creating a self-perpetuating and self-cleaning ecosystem. These methods produce healthier fish, which in turn makes them healthier to eat.

Consumers looking to make a fish purchase that supports this kind of sustainability in aquaculture can choose American-grown fish. As much as 90 percent of the fish we eat comes from other countries, so a purchase of fish produced in the United States supports a smaller carbon footprint as well.

FURTHER READINGS

"Aquaculture." European Commission, European Union. Accessed Jan. 23, 2020. https://ec.europa.eu/fisheries/cfp/aquaculture/aquaculture_methods/history_en

"Aquaculture." Monterey Bay Aquarium Seafood Watch. Accessed Jan. 23, 2020. https://www.seafoodwatch.org/ocean-issues/aquaculture/pollution-and-disease

Carter, Alexandra; and Goldstein, Miriam. "American Aquaculture." Center for American Progress, May 13, 2019. Accessed Jan. 23, 2020. https://www.americanprogress.org/issues/green/reports/2019/05/13/469730/american-aquaculture/

"Does Seafood Have Hormones, Antibiotics, or Drugs?" Seafood Health Facts, NOAA, U.S. Department of Agriculture. Accessed Jan. 23, 2020. https://www.seafoodhealthfacts.org/printpdf/faq/does-seafood-have-hormones-antibiotics-or-drugs

"Farm-Raised Fish." Eat Wisconsin Fish. Accessed Jan. 23, 2020. https://eatwisconsinfish.org/farm-raised-fish/

"Feeds for Aquaculture." NOAA *Fisheries*, Apr. 6, 2018. Accessed Jan. 22, 2020. https://www.fisheries.noaa.gov/insight/feeds-aquaculture

"First-Ever U.S. Tests of Farmed Salmon Show High Levels of Cancer-Causing PCBs." Environmental Working Group, July 30, 2003. Accessed Jan. 24, 2020. https://www.ewg.org/news/news-releases/2003/07/30/first-ever-us-tests-farmed-salmon-show-high-levels-cancer-causing-pcbs

"Fish and Omega-3 Fatty Acids." American Heart Association. Accessed Jan. 23, 2020. http://www.heart.org/HEARTORG/General/Fish-and-Omega-3-Fatty-Acids_UCM_303248_Article.jsp#.XinVJS3MyL4

"Healthy Benefits of Fish." Washington State Department of Health. Accessed Jan. 23, 2020. https://www.doh.wa.gov/CommunityandEnvironment/Food/Fish/HealthBenefits

Hites, Ronald, et al. "Global Assessment of Organic Contaminants in Farmed Salmon." *Science*, Jan. 9, 2004, 303(5655). Accessed Jan. 24, 2020. https://science.sciencemag.org/content/303/5655/226.long

Kendall Reagan Nutrition Center. "Wild Caught vs. Farm Raised Seafood." Colorado State University College of Health and Human Sciences, Apr. 17, 2018. Accessed Jan. 23, 2020. https://chhs.source.colostate.edu/wild-caught-vs-farm-raised-seafood/

Lee, Fan (translated by Ted S.Y. Moo). "Appendix 1: Excerpts from Chinese Fish Culture." Chesapeake Biological Lab, University of Maryland. Original text from 5th century BC. Accessed Jan. 23, 2020. http://www.fao.org/3/ag158e/AG158E04.htm

Leunig, Erich. "Study Identifies Antibiotics in Farm Raised Seafood." Aquaculture North America, Jan. 2, 2015. Accessed Jan. 23, 2020. https://www.aquaculturenorthamerica.com/survey-identifies-antibiotics-in-farm-raised-seafood-1559/

Mikolajczyk, Szczepan, et al. "Farmed Fish as a Source of Dioxins and PCBs for Polish Consumers." *Journal of Veterinary Research*, Sep. 2020. Accessed Apr. 13, 2021. https://www.ncbi.nlm.nih.gov/pmc/articles/PMC7497753/

Murphy, Sean. "Farmed Salmon and Human Health: The Lowdown on PCBs." Seafood Source, July 7, 2015. Accessed Jan. 24, 2020. https://www.seafoodsource.com/news/aquaculture/farmed-salmon-and-human-health-the-lowdown-on-pcbs

National Consumers League staff. "Fish Farms: Good, Bad, or Downright Ugly?" National Consumers League, Aug. 2014. Accessed Jan. 23, 2020. https://www.nclnet.org/fish_farms

"Overview of the U.S. Seafood Supply." Seafood Health Facts: Making Smart Choices. Joint project of Universities of Oregon State, Cornell, Delaware, Rhode Island, Florida, and California, and Community Seafood Initiative. Accessed Jan. 23, 2020. https://www.seafoodhealthfacts.org/seafood-choices/overview-us-seafood-supply

Rabanal, Herminio R. "History of Aquaculture." ASEAN/UNDP/FAO Regional Small-Scale Coastal Fisheries Development Project, Manila, Philippines, 1988. Accessed Jan. 23, 2020. http://www.fao.org/3/ag158e/AG158E00.htm#TOC

Rabanal, Herminio R. "Milestones in Aquaculture Development." ASEAN/UNDP/FAO Regional Small-Scale Coastal Fisheries Development Project, Manila, Philippines, 1988. Accessed Jan. 23, 2020. http://www.fao.org/3/ag158e/AG158E02.htm

"USDA Releases the 2018 Census of Aquaculture Results." National Agricultural Statistics Service, U.S. Department of Agriculture, Dec. 19, 2019. Accessed Jan. 23, 2020. https://www.nass.usda.gov/Newsroom/2019/12-19-2019.php

Fruit and Vegetables Juices

WHAT ARE THEY?

Juice is a drink made by extracting liquid from fruits or vegetables. The term "juice" can also refer to a puree of the edible parts of fruits and vegetables or a concentrate made from the liquid or puree. The FDA requires that beverages containing juice declare the percentage of juice in the formula if their label calls the product juice, if the product has pictures of fruits or vegetables on the label that would lead a consumer to believe there is juice inside, or if "taste and appearance" cause a consumer "to expect juice in the beverage. This includes non-carbonated and carbonated beverages, full-strength (100%) juices, concentrated juices, diluted juices, and beverages that purport to contain juice but contain no juice."

Juices sometimes contain preservatives, which poses the question of whether the contents are indeed 100 percent juice. The FDA states that a product can contain preservatives or other additives and still be 100 percent juice "if the added ingredient does not dilute the juice or, for an expressed juice, change its volume . . . but the percent juice statement must identify the added ingredient, e.g. '100% juice with added preservative.'"

Some juices are labeled as "juice cocktail," a term most often associated with cranberry juice or vegetable juices. These may contain a mix of juices that equal

100 percent juice, but they must specify on the package what the juices are and the percentage of each.

The juice percentage is not required to be on the label if the juice is only a flavoring for a drink, such as a carbonated soft drink, unless the drink uses the word "juice" in the brand name or description (i.e., "juice drink" or "juice beverage"). If the beverage is labeled as "flavored" (i.e., "orange flavored drink"), the juice percentage is not required. Such drinks often contain synthetic flavorings instead of pure juice (see Artificial Flavors earlier in this book).

CURRENT CONSUMPTION STATISTICS AND TRENDS

Research & Markets reported in 2019 that the global juice market reached 45.4 billion liters in 2018. Juice consumption in the United States has dropped from 7.6 gallons per person per year in 2011 to 5.8 gallons per person in 2018. This includes fruit juices, nectars, juice drinks, powdered juices, concentrates, and "others." Fortified juice drinks that contain vitamins, minerals, and antioxidants lead this market, while orange juice is the top seller. At the same time, the trade magazine/website *Beverage Industry* reported in 2019 that juice and juice drink sales have been declining for years in the United States, though trends toward a new juice expression process called high-pressure processing have helped new brands gain ground in the marketplace. This process produces juices that retain more natural ingredients with less sugar, a demand placed on the industry by an increasingly health-conscious public seeking more natural food solutions.

Tropicana Pure Premium leads the juice market in the United States with its orange and grapefruit juices, while leading brands in other juice flavors and blends from May 2018 to May 2019 included Vita Coco, Juicy Juice, Apple & Eve, Capri Sun, and Minute Maid.

NUTRITIONAL INFORMATION

There are many varieties of fruit and vegetable juices, blends, and smoothies, so one set of nutritional figures does not represent them all. In general, however, fruit and vegetable juices contain no saturated fat or cholesterol and often deliver high concentrations of vitamins A and C, as well as smaller amounts of nutrients including calcium and iron.

Fruit juices are among the highest in sugar of all natural foods. An 8-ounce glass of orange juice, for example, contains 112 calories, including 26 g of carbohydrates, of which 21 g is sugar—nearly all the sugar an average adult should have in an entire day.

Vegetable juices, by contrast, are usually made from tomatoes (actually a fruit), carrots, beets, pumpkin, celery, cucumber, spinach, kale, and others. They tend to be lower in calories than fruit juices because they contain a fraction of the sugar that fruit juices do, but they may be high in sodium. A single-serving 8-ounce can of V8 original vegetable juice blend, for example, contains 45 calories and

9 g of carbohydrates, of which 7 g comes from the sugar in the vegetables; it also contains 640 mg of sodium. The low-sodium V8 variety contains 140 mg of sodium. In addition, some vegetable juices contain fruit juice to make them sweeter, which increases the sugar content.

HISTORY

Evidence suggests that people began squeezing fruit to collect its juice as far back as 8000 BC, beginning with grapes for making both juice and wine. The first hard evidence of juice as a commercial product emerged in the sixteenth century in Italy, where the method for making lemonade, a beverage that originated in the Middle East, found its way north. Orange juice followed as much as a century later, and its popularity rose when a book by Scottish doctor James Lind, titled *A Treatise of the Scurvy*, named consumption of citrus fruit as the safeguard against the debilitating illness experienced most often by sailors on long ocean voyages.

The adaptation of the pasteurization method for juice products by Vineland, New Jersey, dentist Thomas Bramwell Welch in 1869 made it possible to store fruit juices without fermenting them. Welch poured grape juice into bottles, sealed them, and then lowered them into boiling water to kill whatever yeast and bacteria might be contained within. This inventive solution made him decide to pursue a career as a drink producer and bottler, providing "Dr. Welch's Unfermented Wine" to consumers. Over time, Welch's company grew to become a top producer of Concord grape juice.

Frozen juice concentrates came to market before World War II, but they were relatively tasteless, as the concentration process removed the fruit's flavor essence along with the water the juice contained. Manufacturers began adding fresh fruit juice to the concentrates before freezing them to replace their flavor, which boosted their popularity but made them more expensive. To stay competitive in the marketplace, makers of frozen juices developed an additive they called a flavor pack, a standardized set of ingredients including the fruit's essential oil, to make certain that every package tastes exactly the same regardless of the relative quality of the fruit, the area from which it was harvested, and the success of that season's crop.

THE CONTROVERSY

The Florida Department of Citrus reports that from July 2018 to June 2019, a wide majority of consumers agreed that orange juice is a healthy choice. Survey data gathered by the global public relations firm Porter Novelli shows that 81 percent of consumers agree that orange juice is healthy and 78 percent say they like the taste of orange juice "a fair amount" or "a great deal." Orange juice continues to have a strong reputation for nutritional value, as 63 percent of consumers believe that 100 percent orange juice is "a great source of vitamins and nutrients."

The survey also collects the opinions of influencers—registered dietitians and others who advise people on healthy eating—and found that 82 percent believe that orange juice is a healthy beverage when consumed in moderation. Notably, no one who took the survey believed that orange juice is unhealthy.

What, then, could be controversial about fruit juices, especially those with "100% Juice" on their labels? Two issues have received media attention in recent years: flavor packs used during processing and the amount of sugar in juice.

To keep up with the enormous demand for fruit juices and to guarantee a consistent quality and taste from batch to batch, many of the leading makers produce the juice, pasteurize it, and store it in large tanks to have it ready for packaging. This juice is processed using a method called deaeration, heating the juice to remove the oxygen and obliterate bacteria before the juice is stored in million-gallon tanks, where it may remain for up to a year. Unfortunately, this process also strips much of the flavor from the juice.

Standardized flavor packs are in use by most major juice processors and bottlers today. Flavor packs are derived from the fruit's peel and pulp, not from laboratory chemicals, so manufacturers are not required by the FDA to call out their ingredients on the juice package's label. Each producer has its own formula for the flavor packs, creating a signature taste that becomes part of that juice's unique brand identity.

"If consumers have the false impression that pasteurized orange juice is not heated or treated because they have a picture of an orange on the carton, then they are not informed," said Kristen Gunter, executive director of the Florida Citrus Growers Association, in an interview with ABC News. "It's not made in a lab or made in a chemical process, but comes through the physical process of boiling and capturing the [orange essence]."

The concept of removing and replacing the juice's taste, however, had some consumers up in arms. In 2012, a group of eight consumers in California filed a lawsuit against Tropicana Products Inc., the nation's leading orange juice company, alleging that the picture of an orange with a straw in it on the Pure Premium juice's packaging, along with the words "all natural," misleads consumers into believing that the juice is fresh-squeezed and unprocessed. In fact, Tropicana's products—like all of the leading juice producers' products—are pasteurized to remove bacteria and increase their shelf life for shipping across the country and beyond. The label tells consumers that the juice has been pasteurized, but it does not mention the addition of flavors after the pasteurization and storage process. The consumers believed that this processing step was in direct conflict with the image on the package, so the carton amounted to false advertising.

Tropicana moved to dismiss the class action suit, but in 2013, a court rejected the company's argument. A recap of the lawsuit through 2016 explained:

> The claims were preempted by the U.S. Food and Drug Administration's rules. U.S. District Judge Dennis M. Cavanaugh [found] that the state regulations at issue were identical to federal regulations, because both state and federal regulations require "accurate and complete labeling of a product's ingredients," including the disclosure of added flavoring.

In July 2019, U.S. district judge William J. Martini dismissed the class action suit, saying that "the labeling on various different products included in the claim were too different, and therefore should be evaluated individually to determine if they were misleading. . . . These variations [in the product labels] are the poster child for lack of predominance." The judge also said that it would be impossible for the plaintiffs to prove that everyone in the class action had been misled by the labeling into purchasing a product they did not know had been processed.

Despite this decision, Tropicana and other juice producers battle multiple lawsuits on a regular basis, most of them stemming from the descriptions of their products on their packaging and in their advertising. The perception of flavor packs as chemical additives—rightly or wrongly—tends to infuriate consumers, especially parents of young children who look for the most natural "clean" foods and ingredients they can find for their families.

One issue that has become inescapable, however, is the large amount of sugar found in most fruit juices and some vegetable juices. This sugar comes from the fruit itself—it is the natural sugar (fructose) found in all fruits, rather than added sugar (sucrose, a combination of fructose and glucose) found in fruit drinks and fruit-flavored carbonated beverages. Many fruit drinks—but not juices—contain sugar produced chemically from corn, which appears in ingredient lists as high-fructose corn syrup (HFCS). Long-established medical science tells us that sucrose and HFCS are major contributors to the increasing obesity epidemic in the United States, which links directly to breast, prostate, uterine, colorectal, and pancreatic cancer, as well as fatty liver disease, kidney disease, high blood pressure, and type 2 diabetes.

Juices do not contain much fiber, as the fiber remains behind after the fruit or vegetable has been squeezed for its juice. Randomized controlled trials that tested the effect on glycemic control of consuming 100 percent fruit juice found that these juices do not increase the risk of diabetes, so they are definitely a better choice than soft drinks loaded with refined sugar. Doctors, dietitians, and researchers agree, however, that just drinking fruit and vegetable juices does not provide the nutritive value of eating whole fruits and vegetables.

Fruit and vegetables provide plenty of fiber, which helps us feel full after a meal and aids in digestive system health, easing bowel movements and slowing the absorption of fat and sugar into the bloodstream. Eating fresh fruit and vegetables is the more effective way to get the benefits of fiber.

FURTHER READINGS

"2019 State of the Beverage Industry: Juice Category Challenged to Maintain Market Share." Beverage Industry, July 15, 2019. Accessed Jan. 26, 2020. https://www.bevindustry.com/articles/92243-2019-state-of-the-beverage-industry-juice-category-challenged-to-maintain-market-share

"A Food Labeling Guide." Food and Drug Administration, U.S. Department of Health and Human Services, Jan. 2013. Accessed Jan. 26, 2020. https://www.fda.gov/media/81606/download

Bedford, Emma. "Per Capita Consumption of Juices in the United States from 2010 to 2018." Statista, Jan. 23, 2020. Accessed Jan. 26, 2020. https://www.statista.com/statistics/257149/per-capita-consumption-of-fruit-juices-in-the-us/

Murphy, Mark, et al. "100% Fruit Juice and Measures of Glucose Control and Insulin Sensitivity: A Systematic Review and Meta-analysis of Randomized Controlled Trials." *Journal of Nutritional Science*, Dec. 15, 2017, 6(59). Accessed Jan. 27, 2020. https://www.cambridge.org/core/journals/journal-of-nutritional-science/article/100-fruit-juice-and-measures-of-glucose-control-and-insulin-sensitivity-a-systematic-review-and-metaanalysis-of-randomised-controlled-trials/75266999F0E7BD2733A3CD4BAD848324

"Florida Citrus Global Marketing Annual Report 2018–2019." Florida Department of Citrus, 2019. Accessed Jan. 27, 2020. https://app.box.com/s/km0jzc0xllxev4lps8codkcbj7o4vdhv

"Global Fruit Juice Market 2018–2019 & Forecasts to 2024 — Focus on 100% Fruit Juice, Nectars, Juice Drinks, Concentrates, Powdered Juice and Others." Research & Markets, Mar. 19, 2019. Accessed Jan. 26, 2020. https://www.prnewswire.com/news-releases/global-fruit-juice-market-2018-2019—forecasts-to-2024—-focus-on-100-fruit-juice-nectars-juice-drinks-concentrates-powdered-juice-and-others-300814856.html

James, Susan Donaldson. "Orange Juice's 'Secret' Flavor Packet Surprises Some Moms." *ABC News*, Dec. 14, 2011. Accessed Jan. 26, 2020. https://abcnews.go.com/Health/orange-juice-moms-secret-ingredient-worries/story?id=15154617

James, Susan Donaldson. "California Woman Sues OJ Giant Tropicana Over Flavor Packs." *ABC News*, Dec. 14, 2011. Accessed Jan. 27, 2020. https://abcnews.go.com/Health/california-woman-sues-pepsicos-tropicana-alleging-deceptive-advertising/story?id=15394357

Milano, Ashley. "Tropicana Orange Juice Class Action Moves Forward." Top Class Actions, May 18, 2016. Accessed Jan. 27, 2020. https://topclassactions.com/lawsuit-settlements/lawsuit-news/335661-tropicana-orange-juice-class-action-moves-forward/

Milne, Iain. "Who Was James Lind, and What Exactly Did He Achieve?" *JLL Bulletin*: Commentaries on the history of treatment evaluation, James Lind Library, 2012. Accessed Jan. 26, 2020. https://www.jameslindlibrary.org/articles/who-was-james-lind-and-what-exactly-did-he-achieve/

"Natural Juice Brands: The History of Juice." Gat Foods. Accessed Jan. 26, 2020. http://www.gatfoods.com/pages/Natural_Juice_Brands_The_History_of_Juice.aspx

"Natural vs. Refined Sugars: What's the Difference?" Cancer Treatment Centers of America, Aug. 9, 2016. Accessed Jan. 27, 2020. https://www.cancercenter.com/community/blog/2016/08/natural-vs-refined-sugars-what-is-the-difference

"Orange Juice: Raw, Nutrition Facts and Calories." SelfNutritionData. Accessed Jan. 26, 2020. https://nutritiondata.self.com/facts/fruits-and-fruit-juices/1971/2

Saner, Emine. "How Fruit Juice Went from Health Food to Junk Food." *The Guardian*, Jan. 17, 2014. Accessed Jan. 26, 2020. https://www.theguardian.com/lifeandstyle/2014/jan/17/how-fruit-juice-health-food-junk-food

Sortor, Emily. "Tropicana Dodges 'Pure' Orange Juice Class Action." Top Class Actions, July 9, 2019. Accessed Jan. 27, 2020. https://topclassactions.com/lawsuit-settlements/consumer-products/beverages/906396-tropicana-dodges-pure-orange-juice-class-action/

Genetically Modified Foods

WHAT ARE THEY?

Genetically modified organisms (GMOs) are animals, plants, or microorganisms within which the genetic material has been changed in a way that would not occur naturally through mating or other acts that combine two or more organisms. The modification takes place at the DNA level, affecting the genetic material of the plant or animal. This process, also referred to as biotechnology, genetic engineering (GE), or gene technology, involves genetic scientists transferring genes from one plant or animal to another to increase, combine, or eliminate specific traits. This can result in a food crop that produces larger and more flavorful products, an animal that becomes resistant to specific diseases, or a bacterium that makes a crop less attractive to pests like locusts.

Food producers find these modifications of interest because they can increase the abundance of a crop, make a fruit or vegetable larger and more attractive to consumers, create a hardier plant that can resist storms or survive drought, or raise herds of cattle that maintain good health and produce more milk. Most genetically modified products currently on the market help crops develop resistance against plant diseases, by making the plant stronger and more tolerant of herbicides and pesticides.

Some plants have been modified by adding a bacterium that makes the plant toxic to the insects most attracted to it. This bacterium, *Bacillus thuringiensis*, is safe for humans, and it greatly reduces the need to spray additional pesticides on crops in the field.

CURRENT CONSUMPTION STATISTICS AND TRENDS

Most GMO crops grown in the United States are fed to animals. Nearly all Americans eat foods that contain genetically modified crops, however: Cornstarch, corn syrup, corn oil, soybean oil, canola oil, and granulated sugar are all listed by the FDA as foods produced from GMO crops including corn, soybeans, canola, and sugar beets. Some fruits and vegetables including potatoes, some forms of squash, apples, and papayas have been modified to increase their resistance to pests and plant diseases. The FDA notes that in 2018, 94 percent of all soybeans planted in the United States had genetic modifications, as well as 92 percent of domestic corn crops. In 2013, 95 percent of canola and 99.9 percent of all sugar beets harvested in the United States came from GMO crops. As the resulting oils, cornstarch, and sugar may be used in thousands of different packaged products as well as in homes, it is likely that just about every American—and everyone worldwide—regularly eats foods that contain GMOs.

The FDA notes that more than 95 percent of domestic animals in the United States eat GMO crops and these animals produce the meat and dairy products we all consume daily. Studies have shown that the modified DNA in the foods these animals eat does not transfer to the animals, so a cow that eats GMO grain does not turn into a GMO animal. "In other words," the FDA explains, "cows do not become the grass they eat and chickens don't become the corn they eat." The GMOs do not transfer into the milk, meat, or eggs consumed by humans.

NUTRITIONAL INFORMATION

No general statement can be made about the nutritional content of all GMO foods.

Gene modification can change the nutritional content of food intentionally: Some canola oil, for example, has been genetically modified to increase the amount of vitamin A it contains. Some modifications may also make unintentional changes to a food's nutritional profile, reducing the amount of one vitamin by increasing another.

HISTORY

Farmers have known for millennia that they can choose the best of their crops and use those seeds to replant the following season, perpetuating a genetic line that produces larger, tastier, and hardier fruits and vegetables. Even before indigenous people moved from nomadic existence to agrarian societies, they bred animals to produce pets—a practice that began some thirty-two thousand years ago, when East Asian hunters encountered wolves that joined them as a pack in hunting for large game. The hunters managed to domesticate these wolves and turn them into companions, encouraging the males to mate with more docile females until they bred themselves a pack of pets. As the practice moved on from one generation to the next over many millennia, breeders learned how to select individuals for their hair length, color, size, body shape, and so on until they had many different and diverse breeds—many of them bearing no resemblance to the original wolves.

Charles Darwin coined the terms "selective breeding" and "artificial selection" in 1859, but by this time, the process had become well established. The first documented use with plants emerged around 7800 BC—this time in the southwestern part of the continent, at the Chogha Golan archaeological site in Iran. Here scientists discovered several varieties of wheat and concluded that the wild forms of the plants had been manipulated to produce new domestic species that would be easier to grow and harvest.

Choosing specimens with the most desirable traits and mating them produced champion race horses, fabulous hothouse flowering plants, and all manner of healthier and more abundant crops. If anyone found this process controversial, they did not leave a record of it—in fact, genetic modification did not become an issue for consumers until the last few decades, when the process moved from choosing the best seeds or the most productive cows to manipulating the genes themselves in a laboratory.

In 1973, two scientists—Herbert Boyer and Stanley Cohen—created the first genetically engineered organism by developing a method to remove a specific gene from one organism and paste it into another one. They transferred a gene that provides antibiotic resistance into a strain of bacteria, making those bacteria resistant to antibiotics. A year later, another pair of scientists, Rudolf Jaenisch and Beatrice Mintz, succeeded in moving foreign DNA into a mouse embryo.

As science celebrated these achievements, however, the media and governments began to object almost immediately. What could the effect of genetic manipulation be on human health? Would this upset the delicate balance of Earth's ecosystems? Should geneticists be playing God?

By mid-1974, the entire world had shut down further research on GE to give experts time to come together and consider the ramifications. They met at the Asilomar Conference of 1975, holding panels of government officials, scientists, and attorneys to discuss the methods, the research, and the potential benefits and threats this new technology posed to life as they knew it. The result was a list of guidelines for the safety of researchers, the containment of each experiment to avoid any negative effects, and the communication stream between researchers around the world as they developed new methods and made additional discoveries.

This extraordinary level of transparency among scientists led to breakthroughs in genetic modification, including the development of patentable organisms that could be marketed by biotechnology companies. In 1992, the U.S. Department of Agriculture approved the first genetically engineered food crop, FLAVR SAVR tomatoes, modified to increase its shelf life and produce a firmer fruit. The FDA followed this in 1995 with approval of a crop that produced its own insecticide. In 2000, Golden Rice, a rice product engineered to increase its vitamin A content, became the first crop produced to reduce nutrient deficiency in underserved populations.

THE CONTROVERSY

Many consumers consider modifications that take place in a laboratory to be suspicious and potentially harmful, as a Pew Research report noted in late 2016. Pew reported that most Americans do not have a working understanding of what GMOs actually are and are "not sure about whether such foods are better or worse for one's health." Just about half the people surveyed said that GMOs had no more effect on human health than any other food, and 10 percent actually said they were probably better for our health. The remaining 39 percent believed that GE of food products actually harms them.

Those who are either skeptical or actually fearful of GMOs tend to base their beliefs on the certainty that scientists have been bought by the industries they serve; the researchers' "desire to help their industries" influences their recommendations on whether a specific GMO is safe to eat. While the scientific community around the world sees GMO foods as no more dangerous than any other food, the idea that anything genetically modified can be dangerous solidified in the 1990s, with the effect of making people's fears very difficult to dispel.

With this in mind, why haven't there been more legal challenges to the use of GMOs? One court case in 2000 demonstrated the federal courts' response to this and the potential for future lawsuits: *Alliance for Bio-Integrity vs. Shalala*. The plaintiff attempted to make the case that GMO foods should be tested the same way that food additives are, because they could have health risks that have not yet revealed themselves in these early days of GMO technology. The complaint continued with the argument that the FDA's decision that GMOs fit the GRAS determination had been spurious and not well considered. The court, however, rejected all of these arguments in favor of the FDA, setting the precedent that cases against GMOs based in popular opinion instead of science would not succeed. This left future plaintiffs with the burden of proof of harm.

The U.S. Supreme Court ruled on its first case involving genetically engineered crops in 2010, overturning a lower court's decision to place an injunction on Monsanto's sale of pesticide-resistant alfalfa seeds until their environmental impact could be researched more fully. The suit, brought by environmental groups, farmers, and consumers, pointed out that Monsanto's alfalfa seed, which had been modified to resist the broad-spectrum herbicide Roundup, could mingle with unmodified seed in fields near the farms using it and create "superweeds" that would not be eradicated by herbicides. The Supreme Court sided with Monsanto in finding the injunction against the company to be a greater measure than necessary. The battle over Monsanto's herbicide-resistant seeds continued beyond this case, however, extending to its sugar beets seed as well; after another battle in the courts, a federal appeals court in California overturned a lower court's order that the entire sugar beet crop be destroyed rather than harvested because it grew from genetically engineered seed. "The Plaintiffs have failed to show a likelihood of irreparable injury," the court's decision said. "Biology, geography, field experience, and permit restrictions make irreparable injury unlikely."

As of 2016, sixty-four countries required mandatory labeling of GMO foods. The United States is not among these, despite calls for such labeling from advocacy groups, but the clamor for this information has encouraged food packagers that do not use GMO ingredients to label their packaging "No GMOs." Advocates argue that consumers should have the option of buying products that do not contain GMOs, whether or not these organisms have any effect at all on the human body. Some restaurant chains—Chipotle and Panera among them—also stock their menus with "clean" foods that contain no GMOs or preservatives.

Not everyone believes that labeling foods that contain GMOs would be good for consumers. Agricultural organizations fear that labeling these foods would cause unnecessary anxiety or aversion to purchasing the products, which would decrease demand for crops like corn and soybeans. Lack of demand would drive up the prices of these products, repelling more consumers and potentially putting companies and farmers out of business.

At the same time, predictions by the United Nations and other organizations focused on world hunger make GMOs more important as the world's population grows. The UN predicts that the world will need to increase food production by 70 percent around the globe by 2050 to feed everyone adequately. Crops that resist disease and pests will become ever more important going forward, leading to larger yields from every field and more food on every table. Crops that provide more nutritional value, like the engineered Golden Rice, may also help world leaders address food shortages in countries facing the negative effects of climate change.

This controversy remains unsettled, though the fact that GMOs have become ubiquitous, especially in processed foods, makes it harder for those opposed to them to pinpoint and prove specific harmful effects.

FURTHER READINGS

"3. Public Opinion About Genetically Modified Foods and Trust in Scientists Connected with These Foods." Pew Research Center, Dec. 1, 2016. Accessed Oct. 8, 2020. https://www.pewresearch.org/science/2016/12/01/public-opinion-about-genetically-modified-foods-and-trust-in-scientists-connected-with-these-foods/

Balter, Michael. "Farming Was So Nice, It Was Invented At Least Twice." *Science*, July 4, 2013. Accessed Oct. 8, 2020. https://www.sciencemag.org/news/2013/07/farming-was-so-nice-it-was-invented-least-twice

"Frequently Asked Questions on Genetically Modified Foods." World Health Organization, May 2014. Accessed Oct. 8, 2020. https://www.who.int/foodsafety/areas_work/food-technology/faq-genetically-modified-food/en/

"GMO Crops, Animal Food, and Beyond." U.S. Food and Drug Administration, Sept. 28, 2020. Accessed Oct. 8, 2020. https://www.fda.gov/food/agricultural-biotechnology/gmo-crops-animal-food-and-beyond

Koons, Jennifer. "Supreme Court Lifts Ban on Planting GM Alfalfa." *Greenwire*, June 21, 2010. Accessed Oct. 8, 2020. https://archive.nytimes.com/www.nytimes.com/gwire/2010/06/21/21greenwire-supreme-court-lifts-ban-on-planting-gm-alfalfa-57894.html

Rangel, Gabriel. "From Corgis to Corn: A Brief Look at the Long History of GMO Technology." Harvard University, The Graduate School of Arts and Sciences, Aug. 9, 2015. Accessed Oct. 8, 2020. http://sitn.hms.harvard.edu/flash/2015/from-corgis-to-corn-a-brief-look-at-the-long-history-of-gmo-technology/

United States Court of Appeals for the Ninth Circuit. No. 10–17719, D.C. No. 3:10-cv-04038-JSW, Feb. 25, 2011. Accessed Oct. 8, 2020. https://web.archive.org/web/20131016004552/https:/articles.law360.s3.amazonaws.com/0228000/228390/monsanto.pdf

Young, Sandra. "Genetically Modified Organisms (GMO)." Discovery Eye Foundation, Feb. 19, 2015. Accessed Oct. 8, 2020. https://discoveryeye.org/gmo-and-nutritional-content-of-food/

Gluten

WHAT IS IT?

Gluten is the substance in foods that helps those foods retain their shape. A set of proteins found in wheat including barley, durum, einkorn, emmer, farina, farro, graham, khorasan wheat, rye, semolina, spelt, triticale, and wheatberries, gluten serves as the glue, holding together baked goods and other products made with one or more of these grains and providing the stretchiness that allows pizza and bread dough their flexibility.

Gluten shows up in a wide range of products, some of which most consumers would not expect. Baked goods, cereals, pasta, and any sauce containing roux (made from butter and flour) are obvious sources of gluten, but soups, salad dressings, sauces in frozen vegetables, imitation meats, malt, food coloring, soy sauce, modified food starch, some vitamin supplements, beer, brewer's yeast, and even toothpaste all may contain gluten as well. Oats are naturally gluten-free, but if the oats grew next to a wheat field, there can be cross-contamination that mixes wheat in with the oats during harvest.

CURRENT CONSUMPTION STATISTICS AND TRENDS

Just about everyone who can tolerate gluten has eaten it at some point in their lives. There are no specific statistics for total gluten consumption, but according to an IndexBox report in 2016, United States consumers ate 16.2 million tons of bread that year, while China consumed 10.2 million tons, Russia 9.6 million tons, and the United Kingdom 6.8 million tons of bread. Germany, Egypt, and Italy also lead the world in bread consumption. Despite most gluten appearing in foods that are simple carbohydrates—which are known for elevating glucose and A1C levels, indicators of diabetes—consumption of these products has seen considerable growth in recent years, and these figures are expected to rise as the world's population continues to expand.

On the other hand, growth in the market for gluten-free products grew an average of 28 percent per year from 2004 to 2011 and is now valued at $4.3 billion globally, with forecasts suggesting it will reach $7.5 billion by 2027. Allied Market Research suggests that the increase in the number of diagnoses of celiac disease and gluten intolerance is fueling this market, but its report also claims that gluten-free products "help improve cholesterol levels, digestive systems, and increase energy levels. Most of the gluten-free foods available are healthy, and help in the weight loss with right combinations and proportions of other foods." These claims are not necessarily borne out by science.

NUTRITIONAL INFORMATION

As many at 1 percent of the world's population has celiac disease, a hereditary autoimmune disorder in which gluten actually damages the small intestine, preventing the absorption of nutrients. This can lead to other serious health issues. Some people have one of several other digestive issues that may require them to eliminate gluten from their diet: non-celiac gluten sensitivity (NCGS), also known as gluten-sensitive enteropathy (GSE); a wheat allergy; or dermatitis herpetiformis (DH), a skin rash from eating gluten.

For the 99 percent of the population that do not have celiac disease or any of the other issues, however, not only is gluten harmless, but it has important positive effects on the body's health.

Gluten works as a prebiotic, acting as nourishment for the good bacteria in the human digestive system. A carbohydrate in gluten derived from wheat bran, arabinoxylan oligosaccharide, stimulates the good bacteria in the colon and helps prevent conditions including inflammatory bowel disease, colorectal cancer, and irritable bowel syndrome.

To date, no scientific studies have shown that eliminating gluten from a healthy person's diet has a beneficial effect. People with celiac disease or another gluten sensitivity are the only population that needs to pursue a gluten-free lifestyle.

If people who have not been diagnosed with celiac disease have symptoms of it—fatigue, bloating, constipation alternating with diarrhea, or more severe issues including unintentional weight loss and malnutrition—they should see a doctor for testing. Undiagnosed celiac disease, NCGS, wheat allergy, or DH are common problems; putting off the diagnosis can lead to intestinal damage that may be permanent.

HISTORY

Physicians have known about celiac disease for thousands of years. The first description of it came from the writings of Greek physician Aretaeus of Cappadocia, who detailed the cases of patients who ate regularly but for whom food passed right through their digestive system without the body taking any nutrition from it. No one made the connection between this mysterious disease and gluten for many centuries.

During World War II in the Netherlands, in a time that came to be known as the Hunger Winter of 1944–1945, a Dutch pediatrician named Willem-Karel Dicke found an opportunity to test a theory he had postulated in the 1930s. That winter, people around him struggled to subsist on 500–1,000 calories a day as the Nazis cut off supplies to the country. He had treated children with celiac disease for decades, but suddenly, when there was no bread to be had throughout the country and four million people began to starve, these children saw their symptoms disappear. Some of them even gained weight, surviving on nothing but the thin broth the soup kitchens could produce.

When the war ended and wheat and bread returned to the country, the children with celiac began to sicken once again. Dicke began a series of experiments with his young patients and found that a wheat-free diet cleared up the children's diarrhea and led directly to weight gain. He shared this information with colleagues, and a team of scientists determined that gliadin, a protein in the wheat gluten, caused the inflammation in the children's bowels.

THE CONTROVERSY

Recent media attention has made many people believe that gluten may not belong in a healthy diet or that it may actually be harmful to otherwise healthy people. The proliferation of grocery products labeled as gluten-free, coupled with the appearance of a gluten-free aisle in many supermarkets, serves as a signal to consumers that there is something wrong with eating food that contains gluten.

A number of movie and television celebrities have chosen a gluten-free lifestyle, whether or not they actually have a medical need for such a diet. Zooey Deschanel, Jessica Alba, Miranda Kerr, Pete Evans, and Lady Gaga are among the luminaries who tout their gluten-free choice. Ryan Phillippe, Victoria Beckham, and Emmy Rossum also tweet and post to Instagram about being gluten-free, but these celebrities actually have celiac disease or a gluten sensitivity.

Just as stars embracing low-carb diets and colon cleanses triggered nationwide enthusiasm for these choices in the 1990s and 2000s, high visibility in Hollywood for gluten-free foods has encouraged many people to try out this lifestyle as well. Whether they can experience any benefits from reducing or eliminating gluten in their diet, however, becomes a separate issue.

According to a 2013 study commissioned by Mintel, 65 percent of American adults tested believed that gluten-free foods were healthier than foods with gluten in them. In the survey of 2,000 adults, 247 people said they ate gluten-free food for reasons other than celiac disease or another sensitivity. In fact, 27 percent chose gluten-free products specifically to assist in weight loss. Mintel analyst Amanda Topper noted,

> It's really interesting to see that consumers think gluten-free foods are healthier and can help them lose weight, because there's been no research affirming these beliefs. The view that these foods and beverages are healthier than their gluten-containing counterparts is a major driver for the market, as interest expands across both gluten-sensitive and health-conscious consumers.

Why do people who do not have one of these conditions turn to the gluten-free diet? Some have symptoms they believe to be related to undiagnosed celiac disease, but that may really indicate something else—for example, lactose intolerance or irritable bowel syndrome. They attempt to self-medicate with a diet rather than see their doctor for an actual diagnosis. If these people do have celiac disease and they have already gone gluten-free before diagnosis, they may eventually want to confirm their condition with a test—but it may be too late to do this. An accurate diagnosis requires the patient to consume gluten regularly before getting tested; without exposure to gluten, the test can return a false-negative result.

Most of the people who choose to go gluten-free expect a resulting weight loss as well as an increase in energy, alertness, and stamina as they eliminate wheat products. To date, no randomized, double-blind, peer-reviewed study has proved that a gluten-free diet will lead to any of these improvements. A retrospective study—one in which participants answered questions about their experiences with various diets—determined that while some respondents who followed a gluten-free diet saw a decrease in weight and an increase in HDL cholesterol over a period of one year, there was no significant difference in frequency of metabolic syndrome or other cardiovascular risk in patients who did not eat gluten. "Lastly, most [gluten-free] followers were health-conscious, well-educated women who may have been predicted to have better cardiovascular profiles than the general population, as well as greater diligence in pursuing weight loss," one reviewer of the study noted.

One questionnaire-based study in 2015 asked 910 endurance-sport athletes without celiac disease if they followed a gluten-free diet and what results they experienced from it. Forty-one percent of those surveyed said that they followed a gluten-free diet more than 50 percent of the time, and more than half of them said they did so because they had self-diagnosed a gluten sensitivity. Of these, 84 percent reported an improvement in their symptoms when they avoided gluten—but they did not report weight loss or performance benefits. A follow-up double-blind study of thirteen cyclists determined that there was no difference in athletic performance between athletes on a gluten-free diet and athletes who ate foods containing gluten.

Maintaining a gluten-free diet without a medical reason can become problematic when we weigh the risks against the benefits. Gluten-free items may contain fewer nutrients or smaller amounts of necessary vitamins than do products containing gluten, providing less fiber, iron, potassium, B vitamins, trace minerals, and zinc than normal breads and pastas. If the individual does not balance this lack of nutrients with other foods that contain these vitamins and minerals, they can risk vitamin deficiencies that can compromise their health. People eating a gluten-free diet are also more likely to choose refined, starchy grains at meals like rice and corn, which can spike glycemic levels, rather than whole grains and fiber like quinoa, lentils, or beans.

Gluten-free products may also cost considerably more: A 2015 study determined that gluten-free bakery products were 267 percent more expensive than gluten-containing goods and gluten-free cereals tended to be more than 200 percent higher priced than normal cereals.

A final word on this from Daniel A. Leffler, MD, director of clinical research at the Celiac Center at Beth Israel Deaconess Medical Center in Boston, in an article in *Harvard Health*: If you choose a gluten-free diet and do not have any kind of gluten sensitivity, it may not be advisable to crow openly about the benefits you may or may not receive from it. More than 300,000 people have no choice but to avoid gluten or risk debilitating illness. "It's a gigantic burden for those who have to follow it," he said. "They get frustrated when they hear how wonderful this diet is."

FURTHER READINGS

Adler, Douglas G. "The Grim Origins of Gluten-Free." *Discover*, Apr. 22, 2019. Accessed Oct. 9, 2020. https://www.discovermagazine.com/health/the-grim-origins-of-gluten-free

"Global Bread and Bakery Consumption Continues to Experience Modest Growth." *FMCG News Global*, Biz Community, Apr. 23, 2018. Accessed Oct. 8, 2020. https://www.bizcommunity.com/Article/1/162/176273.html

"Gluten: A Benefit or Harm to the Body?" *The Nutrition Source*, Harvard T.H. Chan School of Public Health. Accessed Oct. 8, 2020. https://www.hsph.harvard.edu/nutritionsource/gluten/

Jones, Amy L. "The Gluten-Free Diet: Fad or Necessity?" *American Diabetes Association Diabetes Spectrum*, May 2017, 30(3), 118–123. Accessed Oct. 8, 2020. https://www.ncbi.nlm.nih.gov/pmc/articles/PMC5439366/#!po=73.5294

Kale, Raju; and Deshmukh, Roshan. "Gluten-Free Products Market by Type . . . and Distribution Channel: Global Opportunity Analysis and Industry Forecast, 2020–2027." Allied Market Research, Apr. 2020. Accessed Oct. 8, 2020. https://www.alliedmarketresearch.com/gluten-free-products-market

Lis, D.; Stellingwerff, T.; Kitic, C.M.; Ahuja, K.D.; and Fell, J. "No Effects of a Short-Term Gluten-Free Diet on Performance in Nonceliac Athletes." *Medical Science of Sports and Exercise*, 2015; 47(12), 2563–2570. Accessed Oct. 9, 2020. https://pubmed.ncbi.nlm.nih.gov/25970665/

Niland, Benjamin; and Cash, Brooks. "Health Benefits and Adverse Effects of a Gluten-Free Diet in Non-celiac Disease Patients." *Gastroenterology and Hepatology*, Feb. 2018, 14(2), 82–91. Accessed Oct. 9, 2020. https://www.ncbi.nlm.nih.gov/pmc/articles/PMC5866307/#B59

Strawbridge, Holly. "Going Gluten-Free Just Because? Here's What You Need to Know." Harvard Health Publishing, Harvard Medical School, Feb. 20, 2013. Accessed Oct. 9, 2020. https://www.health.harvard.edu/blog/going-gluten-free-just-because-heres-what-you-need-to-know-201302205916

Watson, Elaine. "Health/Weight-Conscious Consumers Are Driving the Gluten-Free Market, Not Celiacs, Says Mintel." Food Navigator-USA.com, Oct. 15, 2013. Accessed Oct. 8, 2020. https://www.foodnavigator-usa.com/Article/2013/10/15/Healthy-eaters-dieters-not-celiacs-propelling-gluten-free-market#

"What Is Celiac Disease?" Celiac Disease Foundation. Accessed Oct. 8, 2020. https://celiac.org/about-celiac-disease/what-is-celiac-disease/

Grains

WHAT ARE THEY?

Grains are the seeds of tall, grassy plants including wheat, rice, corn, barley, oats, sorghum, millet, rye, and other cereal plants. They are included in the diets of virtually every country around the world, providing a cost-effective, easily renewable source of food for humans, livestock, and many wild animals. Grains can be credited with spawning early technologies including mills and the use of water power to run them, and they played a major role in the expansion of civilizations on six continents. Today grains are a key ingredient in many processed foods. Other kinds of ingredients can be produced from grain—corn syrup and corn oil, for example, come from processing corn.

Pseudocereals, a second class of grain-like foods, are not actually grains but provide some similar benefits in a healthy diet. Quinoa and buckwheat are both pseudocereals.

Health professions draw a critical distinction between whole grains and refined grains and their effects on the human diet. Whole grains have three parts: (1) bran, the hard shell of the grain, which contains most of the fiber and minerals; (2) germ, the core of the grain, which holds the proteins, fats, carbohydrates, vitamins, minerals, antioxidants, and other nutrients; and (3) endosperm, which contains starch and protein. When the bran and germ are removed from the grain, only the refined grain (endosperm) remains. Most of the grain humans eat has been refined, removing the fiber, nutrients, and antioxidants and leaving the carbohydrates and some protein. (Many whole grains included in the ingredients of processed foods have been milled into flour, a processing step that defeats their benefits and leaves them similar to refined grains.)

CURRENT CONSUMPTION STATISTICS AND TRENDS

A number of surveys and studies have reached the same conclusion in recent days: Americans know that whole grains are better for them than refined grains. The 2019 Food & Health Survey from the International Food Information Council Foundation, for example, found that of all the foods tested, more people understood that fiber and whole grains are healthful.

Whole grain consumption has increased among adults in the United States, according to the ongoing U.S. Department of Health and Human Services' National Health and Nutrition Examination Survey. From 2013 to 2016, the survey found that 15.8 percent of total grains intake for adults came from whole grains and the percentage increased with age. This demonstrated a significant increase over 2005–2006, when just 12.6 percent of total grain consumption came from whole grains.

At the same time, overall consumption of grains, especially wheat, has declined in the United States, in part because high-profile, low-carbohydrate fad diets like Atkins, South Beach, and keto recommend against consumption of any food containing refined flour. While nearly 85 percent of grain consumption continues to be refined grain products, this does represent a reduction in the popularity of refined grains and in highly processed foods in general.

NUTRITIONAL INFORMATION

Whole grains—especially oats and whole wheat—naturally contain fiber and many nutrients, including B vitamins, iron, copper, magnesium, manganese, phosphorus, selenium, vitamin E, and zinc, as well as many antioxidants and phytochemicals, compounds that play a role in protecting the body from disease, including some cancers. The bran slows down the process of turning starch into glucose, preventing blood sugar spikes and promoting a longer feeling of fullness. Bran's fiber also lowers cholesterol, moves more waste through the intestines, and helps prevent blood clots from forming and leading to heart attack or stroke.

Rice, a staple in the diets of many cultures, may be highly refined (long grain and white rice, white jasmine rice, white basmati rice) or a more intact whole grain (brown rice of any variety; black ["forbidden"], purple, or red rice; or wild rice). Whole grain rice provides fiber, vitamins B_1 (thiamin) and B_6, magnesium, phosphorus, selenium, and manganese. Just as refined bread and cereal grains lose their nutritional value, so do all forms of white rice, which has been stripped of its bran and germ.

Corn in its least refined forms—right off the cob, for example—contains B vitamins and minerals including copper, iron, manganese, magnesium, and zinc, as well as antioxidants including lutein and zeaxanthin, which promote healthy eyes. It also contains a high level of starch, however; half an ear (half a cup of corn) is considered a full portion for people with diabetes.

Food packagers often enrich refined grains with B vitamins, folate, iron, and other vitamins. This does not make them healthy, however: Refined grains contain little beyond simple carbohydrates or carbs that have been separated from their beneficial fiber. These carbs break down quickly in the body and turn from starch to sugar, briefly spiking blood sugar levels. When blood sugar crashes a short time later, the body becomes hungry again and craves more starch and sugar. Eating simple carbs like white bread, cookies, snack chips, and cakes can perpetuate a cycle of overeating, which in turn leads to obesity.

HISTORY

Archaeological field research has revealed that people started eating grain about seventy-five thousand years ago, with western Asia serving as the cradle of this shift in food supply. Einkorn and emmer, two of the "ancient grains" that have emerged as organic crops in recent years, grew along river banks and became the ancestors of today's wheat. In 2009, archaeologists discovered the oldest grain silo ever unearthed, in Dhra, Jordan, in the Middle East. They determined that people used this silo to store grain about eleven thousand years ago and found that it contained bits of barley and an ancient wheat.

Scientists found that people of old ate grain the same way we do: boiling it and adding milk or water, grinding it into flour, and steaming rice to soften it. Once they had mixed water with this flour to make an early form of porridge or gruel, the idea of cooking this over a fire could not have been far off. Bread became the single most widely consumed food in civilizations around the world, a status that has not changed since ancient times. In its current form, with leavening to make it rise, refined flour to make it soft and white, and a machine to slice it, some form of bread remains the single most popular food in every culture.

Grains became the foundation of agrarian societies, allowing civilization to grow and flourish with a ready food supply. The Great Wall of China and the Silk Road, two of the most impressive early achievements in architecture, followed lines of cultivation across continents. The portability of grains allowed the great Roman armies to travel on their stomachs, and Jews in ancient Egypt worked hurriedly to bake flat, unleavened bread to carry with them as they fled into the desert to escape slavery. Historians have argued that the nations that possessed cultivated fields and an abundance of grains had more opportunity to make advances in industry, with their food supplies secure and their farming personnel in place. The role of grains in the world's development cannot be overstated; even today, we can see that countries that do not have this solid foundation in renewable food supply cannot support their own populations.

THE CONTROVERSY

How can something as fundamental as grain not be good for you? It is long established fact that whole grains are a healthier choice than refined grains, and we do not find people attempting to argue that the white flour used in cakes, cookies, and white bread is somehow more healthful than whole grain counterparts. That being said, some proponents of low-carb or no-carb diets believe that any grains—whole or refined—do not belong in the human diet and should be banished from our cupboards and pantries.

Carbohydrates are the starches, sugar, and fiber found in many foods, including fruits and vegetables as well as grains. They represent one of the three macronutrients, the ways that the body gains its primary resources of nutrition and energy. (The other two are protein and fat.) Carbohydrates are a necessary part of a balanced diet, serving as the body's main source of energy; our bodies break down all starchy carbs into sugar, which provides the body's resources for normal functioning of the brain, heart, kidneys, and central nervous system. The carbohydrates found in whole grains are critically important to the body's ability to digest food, expel waste through the colon, and control insulin.

In 1972, cardiologist Robert Atkins wrote a book, *Dr. Atkins' New Diet Revolution*, that has since become the bestselling diet book in the world. The Atkins diet proposed that all carbohydrates should be restricted to just 20 percent of a person's diet, because carbs—all flour-based or sugary foods—led to weight gain and metabolic syndrome, a rise in insulin, cholesterol, blood pressure, and other issues that can eventually lead to heart attack, stroke, and diabetes. The Atkins diet recommended replacing these foods with poultry, fish, meats, cheese, and limited amounts of vegetables—with promises that this counterintuitive proposal would lead to significant weight loss.

This diet does cause people who follow it carefully to lose weight, but the dozens of peer-reviewed studies on this hot topic provide differing results among the investigations. Some see weight loss in individuals who follow a strict low-carb diet, while others produce little or no difference between significant reductions in grain-based foods and other diets that reduce specific sets of macronutrients.

In a study published in 2009 in the *New England Journal of Medicine*, for example, the researchers assigned 811 overweight adults to one of four diets, each with different target proportions of fat, protein, and carbs. They followed these test subjects for two years and found that, after six months, they had all lost about the same amount of weight; after two years, the people on the low-carbohydrate diet had maintained about the same weight loss as the people eating a more normal amount of carbohydrates. (This was also true for differing levels of protein and fat.) Their conclusion: Reduced-calorie diets result in weight loss regardless of whether they emphasize reductions in fat, protein, or carbohydrates.

Halton et al. conducted two 20-year studies of 82,802 women, the results of which were published in 2006 and 2008, examining the relationships between low-carb diets and the risks of heart disease (2006) and diabetes (2008). They found that women who followed low-carb diets that were high in vegetable sources of fat and protein lowered their risk of heart disease by 30 percent and also lowered their diabetes risk by 20 percent. Women who ate low-carbohydrate diets in which the fat and protein sources were meats and cheese, however, did not see any such benefit from this.

A low-carbohydrate diet can be beneficial when combined with an overall regimen of healthy eating, but it can also cause significant problems. While the American Diabetes Association and many other proponents of healthy eating confirm that white flour-based breads, cakes, cookies, and other baked goods and snacks contribute to obesity, diabetes, and heart disease, the human body requires the vitamins, minerals, fiber, and yes, the carbohydrates in whole grains (as well as fruits and vegetables) to maintain good health.

Today's Atkins diet, revised from the original, eliminates grains altogether for people who need to lose more than forty pounds, limiting carbohydrates overall to twenty net carbs (total carbohydrates minus fiber) per day and replacing carbs with proteins and three servings of butter, salad dressing, olive oil, and other "healthy fats." For people who have less weight to lose, a small amount of whole grains may be incorporated into the daily regimen, but carbohydrates should not exceed forty net carbs per day.

Other weight loss diets including the ketogenic (keto) diet, the paleo diet, and eco-Atkins (the vegan version of Atkins) all reduce carbohydrates to a minimum, and the zero-carb diet eliminates all carbohydrates, including fruits and vegetables. No scientific study has found zero-carb to be a healthy or advisable way to lose weight or improve overall health, however.

Science finds little value in demonizing all grains or in blaming all grains for the body's metabolic ills. Some studies support the case for limiting grains in a healthy diet, and many, including the American Diabetes Association, recommend avoiding foods made from refined, processed grains that remove the fiber and protein and leave only the simple carbohydrates. Your results may vary.

FURTHER READINGS

2019 Food & Health Survey. International Food Information Council Foundation. Accessed Oct. 9, 2020. https://foodinsight.org/wp-content/uploads/2019/05/IFIC-Foundation-2019-Food-and-Health-Report-FINAL.pdf

Ahluwalia, Namanjeet, et al. "Contribution of Whole Grains to Total Grains Intake Among Adults Aged 20 and Over: United States, 2013–2016. NCHS Data Brief No. 341, National Health and Nutrition Examination Survey, July 2019. Accessed Oct. 9, 2020. https://www.cdc.gov/nchs/data/databriefs/db341-h.pdf

Bradford, Alina. "Low-Carb Diet Facts, Benefits, and Risks." Live Science, Nov. 12, 2015. Accessed Oct. 11, 2020. https://www.livescience.com/52769-low-carb-diet-facts.html

"Compare Low-Carb Diet Plans: Atkins 20, Atkins 40, and Atkins 100." Atkins. Accessed Oct. 11, 2020. https://www.atkins.com/how-it-works/compare-plans

Gunnars, Kris. "Grains: Are They Good For You, Or Bad?" Healthline, June 4, 2017. Accessed Oct. 9, 2020. https://www.healthline.com/nutrition/grains-good-or-bad

Halton, T.L.; Liu, S.; Manson, J.E.; and Hu, F.B. "Low-Carbohydrate-Diet Score and Risk of Type 2 Diabetes in Women." *American Journal of Clinical Nutrition*, 2008, 87, 339–346. Accessed Oct. 11, 2020. https://pubmed.ncbi.nlm.nih.gov/17093250/

Halton, T.L., et al. "Low-Carbohydrate-Diet Score and the Risk of Coronary Heart Disease in Women." *New England Journal of Med*icine, 2006, 355, 1991–2002. Accessed Oct. 11, 2020. https://pubmed.ncbi.nlm.nih.gov/17093250/

"Rice." The Nutrition Source, Harvard T.H. Chan School of Public Health. Accessed Oct. 9, 2020. https://www.hsph.harvard.edu/nutritionsource/food-features/rice/

Sacks, Frank M., et al. "Comparison of Weight-Loss Diets with Different Compositions of Fat, Protein, and Carbohydrates." *New England Journal of Medicine*, Feb. 26, 2009, 360(9), 859–873. Accessed Oct. 11, 2020. https://pubmed.ncbi.nlm.nih.gov/19246357/

Grass-Fed Beef

WHAT IS IT?

Simply put, grass-fed beef comes from cattle that are fed grass rather than a grain-based feed. This differs from free-range beef in that grass-fed cattle may not be allowed to graze in pastures—they may be fed grass while confined in concentrated animal feeding operations (CAFOs), where they are kept in stalls to restrict their movements and rapidly increase their weight. As the requirements for labeling beef as grass-fed are not clearly defined by the U.S. Department of Agriculture, grass-fed cattle may be given feed that contains foods other than grass.

CURRENT CONSUMPTION STATISTICS AND TRENDS

The grass-fed beef market reached $4 billion in 2015, about 4 percent of the total market for beef in the United States. This includes both domestic beef and meat imported from Australia and other countries.

As much as 75 percent of grass-fed beef—an estimated 1.1 billion pounds annually—may not be labeled as such and may be sold as conventional beef, according to a 2017 report by the Stone Barns Center for Food & Agriculture. This beef may be ground and blended with beef from animals raised in CAFOs. This mingling of grass-fed and conventional beef serves to reduce the fat content of beef sold to supermarkets, fast-food chains, and other restaurants, because grass-fed beef tends to be much leaner than grain-fed beef. When cuts from both kinds of beef are ground together, the result is leaner overall, reducing it below the maximum 30 percent fat content allowed by law.

Consumers buy grass-fed beef in supermarkets and other retail outlets or consume it in restaurants where menus often specify that the chef or a chain's management offers only grass-fed beef. Food service operations (cafeterias) may also purchase grass-fed beef. About 12 percent of purchases are made through direct marketing, both online and at farmers' markets.

NUTRITIONAL INFORMATION

A diet of mostly grass instead of processed animal feed changes the composition of the resulting beef. Not only does grass-fed beef contain fewer calories than beef from grain-fed cattle, but it also contains less monosaturated fat and as much as five times more omega-3 fatty acids, which are known to reduce heart disease risk factors, fight inflammation, improve mental health, fight age-related dementia and Alzheimer's disease, and even help prevent cancer. Grass-fed beef may also be high in CLA, which can lower the risk of type 2 diabetes, heart disease, and cancer.

HISTORY

Until the 1950s, virtually all cattle lived in pastures and grazed on readily available grass. In that decade, however, the U.S. Department of Agriculture (USDA) adjusted its standards for "prime" and "choice" grades of meat, and just 50 percent of all beef produced in the United States made the cut. Consumers demanded more USDA Prime and USDA Choice beef, in an era when a thick, juicy steak on the dining room table represented the epitome of the family's success—and the beef industry worked feverishly to take advantage of that demand.

One of the ways to raise the quality level of beef was to fatten the cattle more, and feeding them with grain turned out to be the fastest way to do this. While a grass-fed steer would be ready for butchering in his fourth or fifth year, a grain-fed steer could be harvested in half that time or even less. Grain, a staple of American diets, grew in abundance and sold cheaply, making it a cost-effective solution for ranchers. They also knew that restricting the animals' movement in feedlots made them gain weight more quickly, but this also spread disease—so the introduction of antibiotics, including penicillin, made it possible to reimagine the cattle ranch with stalls that kept the cattle from wandering and grazing, rapidly increasing their body mass.

The actual term for this is grain-finishing, as cattle in these feedlots actually begin their lives grazing in pastures as calves and young bulls or steers and move to stalls to consume grain for the last 160–180 days of their lives. They gain weight rapidly during this last third of their lives, using the energy of youth to grow to the required size for butchering.

This system seemed to work well, producing the tender, meaty steaks and well-marbled cuts that consumers wanted and gaining higher USDA ratings for more beef. Cattle farms could raise more cattle in less space, expanding their herds to more than 100,000 on many farms. Meat packing operations sprang up near these massive farms, ending the practice of transporting thousands of head of cattle by rail to the major stockyards in Chicago and other cities for butchering.

In 1971, however, as the Soviet Union made a major purchase of grains on the global market for the first time and bad weather in 1972 ruined grain crops around the world, the price of wheat, corn, and soybeans began to rise, climbing steadily until they peaked in 1974. Cattle farmers began to look back at feeding their cattle with grass as the less expensive and more viable solution to maintaining their businesses. The move produced less appealing beef, however, and the trend subsided for nearly two decades; but from 1994 to 1996, commodity prices spiked again. Farmers began to see trends in their futures, from consumer concern for the treatment of animals to the effects of climate change, that could signal the need to turn to other methods of feeding their livestock. As they began to market grass-fed beef for its benefits, studies emerged in the 2000s that found actual, positive health attributes in finishing the cattle on grass, including the boosts in omega-3 fatty acids and antioxidants in the meat.

The demand for grass-fed beef has grown significantly in a very short time. Grass-fed products represented just 1 percent of the total beef market in the United States in 2017, but by 2019, they had carved out a 15 percent share.

THE CONTROVERSY

Whether grass-fed beef actually provides greater health benefits than grain-fed beef remains a well-researched point of contention. A 2010 study published in *Nutrition Journal* examined three decades of research and determined that cattle raised on a grass-based diet produced meat with more omega-3s, more CLA, less saturated fatty acids, and less cholesterol.

A 2011 study published in the *British Journal of Nutrition* conducted a randomized, double-blind dietary intake study of grass-fed versus grain-fed beef consumed by adults for four weeks. The researchers determined that grass-fed beef significantly increased the beneficial long-chain *n*-3 polyunsaturated fatty acids in plasma and platelets, well beyond the levels in people who ate grain-fed beef.

Two studies conducted at Texas A&M University Department of Animal Science, published in 2013, compared the effects of ground beef from grass-fed and grain-fed cattle on risk factors for cardiovascular disease and type 2 diabetes. The result: The grass-fed beef tested contained more of the omega-3 fatty acid, α-linolenic acid (ALA), than the grain-fed beef. ALA may lower the risk of cardiovascular disease and slow down cancer cells' growth rate, making it a particularly valuable part of a healthy diet. Both kinds of beef contain this omega-3, but the study found more of it in grass-fed beef. Conversely, the grass-fed beef contained more saturated fat and trans-fat than the grain-fed beef.

Texas A&M scientists then conducted a randomized crossover trial in which adult men ate both kinds of ground beef for five weeks. They found that older men with mildly elevated cholesterol saw a decrease in the HDL (good) cholesterol from eating grass-fed beef, while men with normal cholesterol levels saw an increase in HDL only from eating grain-fed beef. Neither kind of beef affected the men's LDL cholesterol—but both kinds reduced their insulin levels.

"So, at this point, there is no scientific evidence to support the claims that ground beef from grass-fed cattle is a healthier alternative to ground beef from conventionally raised, grain-fed cattle," author Stephen Smith, PhD, ended his report, discounting the many studies that came before his own.

Despite Texas A&M's findings, the superiority of grass-fed beef over grain-fed became conventional wisdom, borne out by additional studies and laboratory research as well as USDA reports. Current information in the USDA FoodData Central database compares the two ground beef products and finds grass-fed beef to be lower in calories, overall fat, saturated fat, and monosaturated fat, and higher in protein than grain-fed beef. Researchers around the world also acknowledge that the quality and composition of the forage will change the meat—so grass-fed beef from Australia may have a different nutritional breakdown and taste when compared to grass-fed beef from Argentina, Japan, and the United States.

This brings us to the second conundrum: What does "grass-fed" actually mean? Consumers see all kinds of labels on beef products, especially ground beef, in supermarkets as well as on menus in everything from fast-food drive-through lines to upscale restaurants. We may be expected to accept that terms like "pasture-raised," "vegetarian fed," "natural," "USDA Organic," and "no artificial hormones" all mean that the cattle who gave their lives for our consumption spent their days in contentment in open pastures, grazing and socializing with others of their ilk.

The truth, however, can be very different from this mental picture. The USDA does not require on-farm inspection to be certain that cattle are grass-fed, so the methods used to provide the cattle with grass may not be as pastoral as implied.

According to a detailed report by the nonprofit sustainable agriculture organization Stone Barns Center for Food and Agriculture, Bonterra Partners, a consulting firm specializing in sustainable agriculture; and SLM, an investment management firm with ecological farming solutions as its focus, truly grass-fed cattle remain in the pasture throughout their lives and eat grass and other forages and are usually slaughtered at between twenty and twenty-eight months of age (grain-fed cattle are slaughtered at sixteen to twenty-four months). Not all cattle classified as grass-fed spend their lives in pastures, however: Cattle farms have found ways to qualify their cattle as grass-fed while supplementing their diet in other ways to produce fatter animals and more marbled meat. At some of these farms, the cattle remain on pasture but are fed supplemental grain mixtures as well as grass, making them "pasture-raised" but not 100-percent grass-fed. Others finish their cattle in feedlot stalls as if they were grain-fed, but feed them grasses or even pellets made from grasses—but that may contain other fillers like grain by-products.

What difference does it make? Plenty, says the report, because scientific research indicates that grass-fed beef provides many benefits over conventional beef, especially for human health. With its high concentrations of omega-3 and omega-6 fatty acids, antioxidants, and CLAs, it provides important nutrients that also guard against disease. Animals in pastures do not require as much treatment with antibiotics because they are not forced into prolonged close proximity to other cattle and their waste products. This dramatically reduces the incidences of *Escherichia coli* and other bacteria in the beef, making it a safer choice for human consumption.

In 2020, the USDA's Food Safety and Inspection Service (FSIS) revised its guidelines for animal-raising claims on the labels of meat or poultry products. The new guidelines state that meat from animals raised on grass pellets in confined situations cannot be labeled as "100% grass-fed" and that when cattle are fed anything other than grass, this must be defined ("Made from cattle that are fed 85% grass and 15% corn"). To determine which claims can be on the labels, FSIS now requires extensive documentation of the methods used to raise and feed the cattle. Its regulations now state: "As outlined in the guideline, for FSIS to approve these particular claims, animals must be fed only grass or forage, with the exception of milk consumed before weaning. In addition, these animals cannot be fed grain or grain byproducts and must have continuous access to pasture during the growing season until slaughter." This is good news for consumers, as clearer guidelines will reduce ambiguity.

FURTHER READINGS

Cheung, Renee; and McMahon, Paul. "Back to Grass: The Market Potential for U.S. Grassfed Beef." Stone Barns Center for Food & Agriculture, et al., Apr. 2017. Accessed Oct. 11, 2020. https://www.stonebarnscenter.org/wp-content/uploads/2017/10/Grassfed_Full_v2.pdf

Daley, Cynthia A., et al. "A Review of Fatty Acid Profiles and Antioxidant Content in Grass-Fed and Grain-Fed Beef." *Nutrition Journal*, 2010, 9. Accessed Oct. 12, 2020. https://nutritionj.biomedcentral.com/articles/10.1186/1475-2891-9-10

"Food Safety and Inspection Service Labeling Guideline: Documentation Needed To Substantiate Animal Raising Claims for Label Submission." Food Safety and Inspection Service, Dec. 27, 2019. Accessed Oct. 12, 2020. https://www.regulations.gov/document?D=FSIS-2016-0021-4653

Ganzel, Bill. "Beef, Feedlots & IBP." Farming in the 1950s and 60s, Wesset's Living History Farms, 2007. Accessed Oct. 11, 2020. https://livinghistoryfarm.org/farmingin the50s/crops_08.html

"Grass-Fed Beef." U.S. Department of Agriculture FoodData Central, Apr. 1, 2019. Accessed Oct. 12, 2020. https://fdc.nal.usda.gov/fdc-app.html#/food-details/452102/nutrients

Gunnars, Kris. "Grass-Fed vs. Grain-Fed Beef—What's the Difference?" Healthline, Dec. 4, 2019. Accessed Oct. 11, 2020. https://www.healthline.com/nutrition/grass-fed-vs-g+rain-fed-beef

McAfee, S.A.J., et al. "Red Meat from Animals Offered a Grass Diet Increases Plasma and Platelet n-3 PUFA in Healthy Consumers." *British Journal of Nutrition*, Jan. 2011, 105(1), 80–89. Accessed Oct. 12, 2020. https://pubmed.ncbi.nlm.nih.gov/20807460/

Smith, Stephen. "Grass-Fed vs. Grain-Fed Ground Beef: No Difference in Healthfulness." *Beef*, Mar. 25, 2014. Accessed Oct. 12, 2020. https://www.beefmagazine.com/beef-quality/grass-fed-vs-grain-fed-ground-beef-no-difference-healthfulness

Smith, Stephen B. "Ground Beef from Grass-Fed and Grain-Fed Cattle: Does It Matter?" Department of Animal Science, Texas A&M University, Dec. 7, 2013. Accessed Oct. 12, 2020. https://animalscience.tamu.edu/2013/12/07/ground-beef-from-grass-fed-and-grain-fed-cattle-does-it-matter/

Green Tea

WHAT IS IT?

All kinds of tea, except for herbal teas, come from the dried leaves of *Camellia senensis*, an evergreen shrub that originated in East Asia. Most teas are made from this shrub's oxidized leaves—the leaves begin to wilt and darken just after they are harvested—so black, oolong, chai, and Earl Gray are darker in color and have a stronger flavor. Enzymes in *C. sinensis*'s chemistry cause the leaves to lose their chlorophyll and release tannins as they dry. Lighter-colored white and yellow teas are made from unoxidized leaves. Green tea comes from the freshest, unwilted leaves before they have a chance to oxidize, allowing it to capture the chlorophyll and produce a leafy green color.

CURRENT CONSUMPTION STATISTICS AND TRENDS

In the $2.58 billion U.S. specialty tea category, green tea represents about 15 percent or $387,000,000 in annual consumption, according to 2019 statistics from the Tea Association of the USA. Favored by a younger audience over black tea and other beverages, green tea is a top choice of millennials, with up to 87 percent drinking tea in general; tea's popularity with this demographic has led coffee shop chains, restaurants, and specialty sections of grocery stores to feature green tea on menus and store shelves and to produce novelty drinks with green tea as a prominent ingredient.

Analysts project major growth for the global green tea market, with green tea bags as a major driver. In the United States, forecasted growth may be as much as nearly 5 percent annually to 2025, and Germany and Japan are expected to see significant growth as well.

NUTRITIONAL INFORMATION

Green tea has no calories, making it a welcome alternative to sugary drinks like carbonated beverages and juices. It contains antioxidants called polyphenols, which help reduce inflammation throughout the body and protect cells from damage, making it a potential defense against the rapid cell growth of cancer. In fact, research indicates that women who drink green tea have a lower risk of developing breast cancer, while men who drink green tea may be less likely to develop prostate cancer. The tea also appears to help prevent colorectal cancer, according to no less than twenty-nine studies that showed a roughly 42 percent decrease in cancer risk among green tea drinkers.

These antioxidants promote strong bones and prevent bone loss, helping to reduce fracture risks in people with osteoporosis. The tea also provides an amino acid called L-theanine, which has the ability to produce a sense of calm—and when combined with the tea's natural caffeine, it improves cognitive performance and alertness and even boosts mood.

Studies have shown that green tea prevents angiogenesis, the formation of new blood vessels required for new fat tissue or cancerous tumors to grow. This can actually help keep a person from gaining weight when used along with a healthy diet. This tea supports the body's immunity by boosting antibacterial, antifungal, and antiviral systems—and it provides prebiotic benefits for healthy gut bacteria as well. Some studies indicate that green tea can be a tool in controlling fasting blood sugar levels, which can be important in preventing diabetes.

HISTORY

Written records from as far back as the Han Dynasty in China (AD 206–220) make mention of the cultivation and drinking of green tea as a medicine for a number of illnesses. Sometime during the Tang Dynasty (600–900), people began drinking green tea simply because they enjoyed it, drying the leaves and compressing them into cakes to make them easy to carry. A groundbreaking book from that era, *The Classic of Tea (Cha Jing)* by Lu Yu, first considered green tea as a culture unto itself and explored all aspects of its use. In the same period, ritual tea ceremonies came into being, elevating green tea drinking to high art among the cultural elite. Drinking green tea, then, became a sign of elevated status, a privilege for the wealthy and powerful.

Centuries passed before green tea found its way into Western civilization. In the late nineteenth century, fast ships allowed merchants to transport green tea leaves quickly enough to reach western Europe and the Americas before they oxidized and became black tea. Once the tea and its many healthful properties became known in the west, its popularity increased, and the exotically colored, surprisingly fresh-tasting brew became part of Western culture. In more recent years, matcha—made by grinding the fresh leaves into powder—has become a staple in coffee shops and an ingredient in baked goods and other confections, and specialty drinks containing green tea are popular from independent coffee/tea shops to Starbucks and Wal-Mart.

THE CONTROVERSY

A 2010 literature review of all the studies of green tea's benefits to that date numbered 105 different credible studies in English alone, making this drink one of the most carefully and thoroughly researched of all the foods in this book. The consensus of these laboratory studies, according to reviewers Sabu M. Chacko et al., is that the catechin (antioxidant) that occurs naturally in green tea showed benefits against obesity caused by a high-fat diet, type 2 diabetes, and coronary disease. In all of these cases, however, laboratory animals received more green tea on a daily basis than any human would be likely to drink.

With all the benefits attributed to green tea—from slowing the aging process to staving off cancer—why isn't everyone drinking it?

It turns out that green tea can have a downside, especially if people drink it daily in great quantities. Researchers also disagree on the amount of green tea people must consume to obtain its beneficial effects, with some espousing just a single cup a day and some requiring five cups or more.

Despite its herbal color and fresh flavor, green tea contains as much caffeine as any cup of black tea, making it a stimulant less powerful than coffee but potent nonetheless. Drinking several cups throughout the day can produce the same issues as coffee: the increased anxiety, headache, restlessness, and difficulty sleeping that all-day coffee drinkers experience.

Takabayashi et al. (2004) noted that consuming large amounts of green tea sometimes caused damage to the liver and pancreas of hamsters in a laboratory. Yun et al. (2006) found that one of the tea's catechins actually acts as a pro-oxidant instead of an antioxidant, producing exactly the opposite effect on high blood sugar and pancreatic functioning to the one desired. Two more studies (Sakamoto et al., 2001; Satoh et al., 2002) found that giving rats a high dose of green tea extract—5 percent of their diet—for thirteen weeks caused their thyroid to enlarge by modifying the plasma concentrations in thyroid hormones. "However, drinking even a very high dietary amount of green tea would be unlikely to cause these adverse effects in humans," the study concluded.

Green tea, like many tea plants, can contain significant amounts of aluminum obtained from the soil in which it grows. This can be harmful to patients who have kidney failure: Normal kidney functioning carries the aluminum out of the body in the urine, but malfunctioning kidneys can allow aluminum to accumulate in the body, which can lead to neurological problems. The tea's catechins may have the opposite effect on iron, drawing this important mineral out of the food a person consumes and carrying it out in urine. This can decrease the amount of iron the body acquires from diet, creating an iron deficiency.

The quality of the tea itself affects its healthful benefits, noted Yi Lu et al. (2004) in a study that tested 12 brands of tea for fluoride content. Many tea plants accumulate fluoride as they grow, and the study found that the more fluoride a plant's leaves contained, the fewer antioxidants it produced. Tea brands known for higher quality contained less fluoride and more antioxidants.

Finally, some studies indicate that adding cow's milk to the tea diminishes the antioxidants in it, a phenomenon that may be related to the amount of fat in the milk. (So far, no research has been conducted using soy, almond, or other plant milk products in green tea.)

Until recently, no studies offered a definitive answer to the question of how much green tea produces either the positive or negative effects in humans. A cohort study conducted in Japan and published in 2020 in *BMJ Open Diabetes Research and Care* (Komorita et al.), however, provided the most information to date about how much green tea is enough to make a difference in a person's health. The study followed 4,923 patients with type 2 diabetes for five years and found that drinking one cup of green tea every day produced a 15 percent lower risk of mortality compared with people who did not drink green tea. Those who drank two or three cups daily saw a 27 percent reduction in risk, and people who drank four or more cups every day saw a 40 percent drop in their risk for mortality. Drinking coffee also produced a lower risk—and people who drank two or more cups of green tea and two or more cups of coffee throughout the day lowered their mortality risk by 51 percent.

"To date, no study has investigated the combined effect of green tea and coffee consumption on all-cause mortality," the researchers wrote. "The present study determined that combined higher green tea and coffee consumption markedly reduced mortality. Further, this cohort study included potential confounders, such as sleep duration, diabetic complications, lifestyle, physical activity, laboratory data, and medications." This study did not note whether the green tea and coffee consumed by the subjects contained caffeine, though decaffeinated coffee and tea are scarce in Japan.

FURTHER READINGS

Bolton, Dan. "Green Tea Market Expected to Grow." *World Tea News*, Dec. 9, 2019. Accessed Oct. 12, 2020. https://worldteanews.com/market-trends-data-and-insights/green-tea-market-expected-to-grow

Komorita, Y., et al. "Additive Effects of Green Tea and Coffee on All-Cause Mortality in Patients with Type 2 Diabetes Mellitus: the Fukuoka Diabetes Registry." *BMJ Open Diabetic Research and Care*, Oct. 21, 2020, 8(1). Accessed Oct. 25, 2020. https://drc.bmj.com/content/8/1/e001252

Lu, Yi; Guo, Wen-Fei; and Yang, Xian-Qiang. "Fluoride Content in Tea and Its Relationship with Tea Quality." *Journal of Agriculture and Food Chemistry*, 2004, 52(14), 4472–4476. Accessed Oct. 13, 2020. https://pubs.acs.org/doi/10.1021/jf0308354

McDonell, Kayla. "How Much Green Tea Should You Drink Per Day?" Healthline, Oct. 3, 2017. Accessed Oct. 12, 2020. https://www.healthline.com/nutrition/how-much-green-tea-per-day#TOC_TITLE_HDR_2

Ryan, Lisa; and Petit, Sébastien. "Addition of Whole, Semiskimmed, and Skimmed Bovine Milk Reduces the Total Antioxidant Capacity of Black Tea." *Nutrition Research*, Jan. 2010, 30(1), 14–20. Accessed Oct. 13, 2020. https://pubmed.ncbi.nlm.nih.gov/20116655/

Sakamoto, Y.; Mikuriya, H.; Tayama, K.; Takahashi, H.; Nagasawa, A.; Yano, N.; Yuzawa, K.; Ogata, A.; and Aoki, N. "Goitrogenic Effects of Green Tea Extract Catechins by Dietary Administration in Rats." *Archives of Toxicology*, 2001, 75, 591–596. Accessed Oct. 13, 2020. https://pubmed.ncbi.nlm.nih.gov/11808919/

Sass, Cynthia. "10 Health Benefits of Green Tea, According to a Nutritionist." Health.com, Aug. 27, 2019. Accessed Oct. 12, 2020. https://www.health.com/food/benefits-green-tea

Satoh, K.; Sakamoto, Y.; Ogata, A.; Nagai, F.; Mikuriya, H.; Numazawa, M.; Yamada, K.; and Aoki, N. "Inhibition of Aromatase Activity by Green Tea Extract Catechins and Their Endocrinological Effects of Oral Administration in Rats." *Food and Chemical Toxicology*, 2002, 40, 925–933. Accessed Oct. 13, 2020. https://pubmed.ncbi.nlm.nih.gov/12065214/

Takabayashi, F.; Tahara, S.; Kanerko, T.; and Harada, N. "Effect of Green Tea Catechins on Oxidative DNA Damage of Hamster Pancreas and Liver Induced by N-nitrosobis (2-oxopropyl) amine and/or Oxidized Soybean Oil." *Biofactors*, 2004, 21, 335–337. Accessed Oct. 13, 2020. https://pubmed.ncbi.nlm.nih.gov/15630222/

"Tea 101: What Is Green Tea?" Art of Tea. Accessed Oct. 12, 2020. https://www.artoftea.com/blogs/tea-101/what-is-green-tea

Yuetong Chen, et al. "An Inverse Association Between Tea Consumption and Colorectal Cancer Risk." *Oncotarget*, June 6, 2017, 8(23), 37367–37376. Accessed Oct. 13, 2020. https://pubmed.ncbi.nlm.nih.gov/28454102/

Yun, S.Y.; Kim, S.P.; and Song, D.K. "Effects of (-)-Epigallocatechin-3-gallate on Pancreatic Beta-cell Damage in Streptozotocin-Induced Diabetic Rats." *European Journal of Pharmacology*, 2006, 541, 115–121. Accessed Oct. 13, 2020. https://pubmed.ncbi.nlm.nih.gov/16765345/

Guar Gum

WHAT IS IT?

Guar gum comes from the guar bean (*Cyamopsis tetragonoloba*), a legume grown and harvested for this purpose. The endosperm of this bean—what's left when the shell and seed are removed—is milled to a powder for use as a bonding substance in food products. It contains a polysaccharide called galactomannan, a combination of two sugars (galactose and mannose), which can absorb water, thicken, emulsify, and turn into a gel. When used as a food additive, it binds together elements that otherwise may not mix.

CURRENT CONSUMPTION STATISTICS AND TRENDS

Found in a wide range of foods including ice cream, yogurt, kefir, juices, pudding, soups, processed cheeses, salad dressing, gluten-free baked goods, cereals, canned and bottled gravy, and others, as well as nonedible products like cosmetics, guar gum plays a significant role in the food industry. Sales of this additive are expected to reach $1.15 billion in 2022, with annual growth of 7.9 percent. Much of this is in the oil well industry, however, which depends on guar gum's gelling ability as a polymer, rather than in food.

On the consumables side, bakery and confectionary manufacturers use the most guar gum for products like gummy candies, jelly beans, marshmallows, fruit leather, caramel, fondant, and flavored fillings.

NUTRITIONAL INFORMATION

By itself, guar gum does not have much nutritional value. It is low in calories and provides a little protein and soluble fiber, both of which can be a benefit to the human body.

HISTORY

How exactly the guar bean became a domestic crop remains a little fuzzy in agricultural history, though historians who have weighed in on the subject believe that it developed from a wild species, C. *senegalensis*, found on the African continent. Arab trades brought the wild bean to southern Asia to feed their horses, arriving there over the course of AD 800s through 1200s, and agrarians in India and what is now Pakistan embraced the bean as a crop. They used it as a food for animals, but milled it for humans as well.

Not until the twentieth century did guar beans make their way west, arriving in the United States shortly before World War I for use in fertilizing crops. In the 1940s, paper and textile manufacturers depended on locust bean gum for industrial applications, importing it from Europe and North Africa, but during World War II, imports became difficult and supplies flagged. The U.S. Department of Agriculture and the Institute of Paper Chemistry began looking in earnest for a readily available substitute and determined through testing at the University of Arizona that guar gum would fit the bill. After the war, in 1948, scientist R.L. Whistler studied guar gum at Purdue University and found that it could have many applications in industry. He recommended that it be grown in the United States for domestic use.

Since Whistler, guar gum gives paper towels their ability to retain their strength and cohesion when wet, and the oil and gas industry uses it to stimulate its wells. It thickens dyes used in cloth and carpets, creates water resistance in dynamite, and encourages slurry explosives to gel. Its use in food products came about more recently, where it prevents the formation of ice crystals in frozen foods, thickens and stabilizes thick liquids and soft solids like ice cream, sauces, and cheese spreads, and adds viscosity to dressings and gravies.

THE CONTROVERSY

The FDA places guar gum in its GRAS category, which means that when used in the ways intended, there are no known harmful effects of adding the substance to foods. Indeed, the science bears this out: Guar gum used in low concentrations (0.5–1 percent of the weight of the total product) moves through the large intestine without incident, comfortably digested by the bacterium *Clostridium butyricum* in the intestinal tract.

Guar gum's fiber content becomes a nutritional asset when partially hydrolyzed (mixed with water), lowering the gum's viscosity and making it easier to mix with various food products to increase their fiber content—without changing the taste or texture of the food. In this form, guar gum can help decrease the symptoms of irritable bowel syndrome. It also decreases the digestion of starch, by serving as a barrier between starch and the enzymes that hydrolyze it in the digestive tract. As guar gum absorbs water within the digestive system and gels, it has the effect of lowering LDL cholesterol and glucose while promoting a feeling of fullness, which helps encourage weight loss and prevent obesity.

Some people may find that eating food with guar gum as an additive produces gas, cramps, bloating, or diarrhea, but this is not the norm. A tiny fraction of people may be allergic to it as well, though the cases that appear in research endured exposure to guar gum powder in manufacturing sites over periods of years.

This is all well and good, as long as the limits on guar gum in food manufacturing are followed and respected—and today's producers of packaged products do exactly this. They learned from the lesson of 1990, when a weight loss product called Cal-Ban 3000, distributed by Health Care Products, Inc., used large amounts of guar gum in its pills in an attempt to cause rapid weight loss.

The gum in Cal-Ban 3000 did what guar gum does: It reached the stomach, combined with water, and swelled up, usually increasing in size by ten to twenty times. This certainly filled the stomach and intestines and created a sense of fullness and a reduction in appetite, though patients did not necessarily lose weight. The outsized portion of guar gum did not stop there, however: It became an obstruction in the small intestine and even the esophagus, backing up the entire digestive system. In seventeen cases, people's throats filled with expanded guar gum; ten ended up in the hospital, and one of them died when a blood clot that formed during surgery to remove the blockage reached a lung.

Florida became the first state to put a stop to the use of Cal-Ban 3000 when it received reports of fifty people within the state who were injured by the drug. A federal court in Tampa issued a restraining order prohibiting Health Care Products from selling the drug, and the FDA quickly stepped in and banned it entirely.

Such a tragedy cannot happen with the carefully regulated amounts of guar gum in our food today. The FDA set maximum levels for the addition of guar gum to food products, allowing just 0.35 percent of total weight in baked goods and up to 2 percent in vegetable juices (that's 4.8 g in a one-cup serving). Continued research has shown that as much as 15 g of guar gum in a serving of food can be used safely, but the FDA exercises an abundance of caution, setting limits that produce the desired effect in food without endangering any consumer's health.

FURTHER READINGS

"Guar Gum Market." Markets and Markets. Accessed Oct. 13, 2020. https://www.marketsandmarkets.com/Market-Reports/guar-gum-market-177796677.html

Kanerva, L., et al. "Occupational Allergic Rhinitis from Guar Gum." *Clinical Allergy*, May 1988, 18(3), 245–252. Accessed Oct. 13, 2020. https://pubmed.ncbi.nlm.nih.gov/3396193/

Lagler, F., et al. "Occupational Asthma Caused by Guar Gum." *Journal of Allergy and Clinical Immunology*, Apr. 1990, 85(4): 785–790. Accessed Oct. 13, 2020. https://pubmed.ncbi.nlm.nih.gov/2324416/

Link, Rachel. "Is Guar Gum Healthy or Unhealthy? The Surprising Truth." Healthline, Sept. 27, 2019. Accessed Oct. 13, 2020. https://www.healthline.com/nutrition/guar-gum

Mesce, Deborah. "FDA Says Don't Use Cal-Ban 3000." Associated Press, July 27, 1990. Accessed Oct. 13, 2020. https://apnews.com/article/ea5ff0f4fd1caca26d9bca163721aad8

Mudgil, Deepak, et al. "Guar Gum: Processing, Properties and Food Applications." *Journal of Food Science and Technology*, Mar. 2014, 51(3), 409–418. Accessed Oct. 13, 2020. https://www.ncbi.nlm.nih.gov/pmc/articles/PMC3931889/#!po=6.00000

Olive Oil

WHAT IS IT?

Just as its name implies, olive oil is a liquid fat cold-pressed from whole olives. It can be purchased in many different varieties and from a number of olive cultivars, but the most popular tends to be extra virgin olive oil, which has the lowest "free acidity," or percentage of fatty acids, at 0.8 percent. Extra virgin olive oil, the one most often used in cooking, comes from young green olives, giving the oil a lighter flavor and texture. It is often served at table for bread dipping and mixing with vinegar for salad dressing.

CURRENT CONSUMPTION STATISTICS AND TRENDS

In 2019, olive oil consumption in the United States reached 362,000 metric tons, which was slightly less than the record-breaking 2018 consumption of 364,000 metric tons. These figures represent major growth since 2000, when

Americans consumed just 209,000 metric tons of olive oil. Global production topped out at 3.12 million tons in the 2019–2020 crop year, though the decrease in production created by the global pandemic in the 2020–2021 agricultural year was expected to see that figure drop to 3.03 million tons in 2021.

NUTRITIONAL INFORMATION

Olive oil is a healthy fat—it contains no protein or carbohydrates (starch or sugar), and its fat content comes almost entirely from heart-healthy oleic acid, an omega-9 monounsaturated fat—9.9 g per tablespoon, which has been shown in peer-reviewed studies to reduce inflammation and even may suppress the growth of some cancer cells. Oleic acid is a nonessential fatty acid, a fat that does not occur naturally in the human body and must be acquired from outside sources, that is, food.

It also contains much smaller amounts of polyunsaturated fat (1.4 g) and saturated fat (1.9 g), which the body needs to absorb vitamins A, D, E, and K from other foods. This combination of factors makes olive oil an important part of a healthy diet. One serving (a tablespoon) of olive oil provides 119 calories and a total of 13.5 g of fat.

HISTORY

"And thou shalt command the children of Israel, that they bring thee pure oil olive beaten for the light, to cause the lamp to burn always," reads Exodus 23:11 in the *King James Bible*, one of the earliest mentions of olive oil in recorded history. While we cannot be sure exactly when these words were written, inventory logs from ships that sailed the Mediterranean Sea as far back as 4000 BC note olive oil in their cargo. By 2500 BC, the oil had become so central to civilization that the Code of Hammurabi codified its trade, setting down rules for its production as well.

In the last millennium BC, the Roman Empire's troops carried olive trees to plant wherever they achieved another victory by conquering the local territory. The Romans, ever resourceful and forward-thinking, had already made many advancements in cultivating olive trees, pressing the fruit to extract the oil, and keeping it fresh in long-term storage. By this time, olive oil's value in every part of the Roman existence made it an acceptable payment in lieu of cash for taxes. When the empire fell in AD 500, olive cultivation declined sharply for a period as some regions lost population and wealth.

Hundreds of years would pass before the Italian olive groves recovered and began to flourish. Tuscany gained a reputation for the quality of its olives and its ability to cultivate varieties of trees. By the fifteenth century, as the Renaissance took hold across Europe, Italy rose to become the largest producer of olive oil in the known world. Noblemen and royalty paid top dollar for Italian olive oil, and merchants developed shipping routes to bring it to far-off consumers.

As the massive wave of immigration crossed the Atlantic Ocean in the 1800s and Italian and Greek immigrants arrived by the thousands in the United States, they introduced the flavors of olive oils to America. Soon the continents across the sea became enthusiastic markets for imports of the oil so many expatriates missed. Demand increased steadily over the years until today, when the quality and variety of olive oils approaches the scope of fine wines, with price points ranging from very affordable, flavorful oils under $10.00 per quart to some 32-ounce bottles that go for more than $100.00.

THE CONTROVERSY

The question of whether olive oil is good for you seems on the surface to be settled science, but this has not stopped some doubters from pursuing the opposite argument: that olive oil, which by definition contains several kinds of fat, must actually be harmful to the point of leading directly to atherosclerosis and cardiovascular disease.

As an important source of oleic acid, olive oil plays a key role in the Mediterranean diet recommended by primary care physicians, professional dieticians, and cardiologists for its remarkable ability to control body weight and maintain optimal health. Oleic acid—also obtainable from avocado oil and macadamia nuts—promotes the reproduction of a cell molecule that keeps cancer proteins from developing and interferes with pathways between cells that allow cancer cells to reproduce. It also helps reduce the decline of cognitive function in older adults and may be part of the solution for preventing or slowing the progress of Alzheimer's disease. Oleic acid reduces inflammation in the body, which can help control the release of insulin to increase blood glucose, making it a good choice for people with type 2 diabetes.

A plethora of studies, including Terés et al. (2008) and Sergio Lopez et al. (2010), have shown that olive oil's high oleic acid content supports the lowering of blood pressure and better cardiovascular health. The research findings have been consistent enough that the FDA determined in November 2018 that they provide "credible evidence to support a qualified health claim that consuming oleic acid in edible oils, such as olive oil, sunflower oil, or canola oil, may reduce the risk of coronary heart disease." The FDA qualified its decision further, saying that the studies have put forward "supportive but not conclusive scientific evidence . . . that daily consumption of about 1½ tablespoons (20 g) of oils containing high levels of oleic acid, when replaced for fats and oils higher in saturated fat, may reduce the risk of coronary heart disease." These oils should not increase the consumer's total number of daily calories, the statement continued—rather, the oils containing oleic acid should replace oils (or butter) with saturated fats.

Here, however, is where doubters target their criticism. Many of them refer to a study (Vogel, 1999) that measures flow-mediated dilation (FMD), or changes in the diameter of the brachial artery in the upper arm, using ultrasound. In this study, researchers looked for the behavior of endothelial cells in the artery, the cells that line all blood vessels throughout the body and are involved in blood clotting, new blood vessel building, and the body's immune system response. These cells produce nitric oxide to expand the blood vessels and keep platelets from gathering on artery walls and forming blood clots. The FMD test measures this expansion.

When a person smokes a cigarette, eats a fatty meal or a sugary dessert, or consumes a lot of salt, FMD becomes impaired and arteries do not dilate normally. This becomes a chronic condition when someone has high cholesterol or diabetes. The 1999 study tested olive oil's effect on FMD against a meal of a hamburger and French fries or a piece of cheesecake. The result: Olive oil caused the same three-hour decline in FMD that these high-fat choices did. Vogel returned to this topic the following year and conducted a new study with ten subjects, feeding them meals with different sources of fat, and found that the meal containing olive oil reduced FMD by 31 percent, more than meals containing canola oil or salmon. He concluded that the Mediterranean diet works to guard against heart disease in spite of its inclusion of olive oil, not because of it.

An often-misquoted 2007 study (Rueda-Clausen et al.) used a randomized controlled trial to reach a similar result, but only compared olive, soybean, and palm oils and their endothelial function. This study acknowledged the overall healthfulness of choosing oils with unsaturated fatty acids like oleic acid, but examined the transformation of these oils in the deep-frying process and its effect on the reaction of the endothelial cells. The study determined that using the oils to deep-fry food did not increase the adverse reaction of the cells. This is not exactly a condemnation of olive oil or any of the others; it simply stated that "all the vegetable oils, fresh and deep-fried, produced an increase in the triglyceride plasma levels in healthy subjects."

A literature review and meta-analysis of thirty such studies, performed in 2015 by Schwingshackl et al., came to the opposite conclusion about olive oil and endothelial response: "These results provide evidence that olive oil might exert beneficial effects on endothelial function as well as markers of inflammation and endothelial function, thus representing a key ingredient contributing to the cardiovascular-protective effects of a Mediterranean diet." The researchers recommended a "conservative approach," stopping well short of declaring olive oil as the solution to cardiovascular health, but acknowledged olive oil's ability to decrease C-reactive protein and interleukin-6, both markers of inflammation somewhere in the body, in comparison to controls.

If olive oil's role in cardiovascular health were not enough to convince people to use it in their daily diet, solid research makes the case for the possibility that eating olive oil may be good for people who have a genetic predisposition to some kinds of breast cancer.

A team of researchers at the Breast Cancer Translational Research Laboratory at Northwestern Healthcare Research Institute in Evanston, Illinois, took on this question in 2005. They used a long list of testing and imaging methods—"flow cytometry, western blotting, immunofluorescence microscopy, metabolic status (MTT), soft-agar colony formation, enzymatic in situ labeling of apoptosis-induced DNA double-strand breaks (TUNEL assay analyses), and caspase-3-dependent poly-ADP ribose polymerase (PARP) cleavage assays"—to perform a thorough analysis of the effects of oleic acid on the Her-2/neu oncogene, one of the most active breast cancer genes. Their conclusion: The oleic acid in olive oil does indeed suppress the development of the gene, "promoting apoptotic cell death of breast cancer cells." Individual fatty acids can help to regulate breast cancer cells, opening up the possibility that olive oil may be a critically important food to include in the diet of a person who carries this breast cancer gene.

More recently, a study published in August 2019 by researchers at Hunter College determined that extra virgin olive oils that contain high concentrations of oleocanthal, an antioxidant with anti-inflammatory properties, actually killed cancer cells in a laboratory. They engineered mice to develop pancreatic cancer, then injected them with oleocanthal, and found that the injection actually shrank their tumors and extended their lifespan by about four weeks—the equivalent of ten human years. No studies have been conducted on human beings yet. "Whether oleocanthal can be used as a magic bullet to target cancer cells is not clear," said David Foster, PhD, the lead scientist for the study. "However, the data provided in this article validated studies indicating that extra virgin olive oil can prevent cancer."

If all of these findings turn out to have merit and validity in the long run, olive oil may rise to the top of the so-called superfoods list, providing a tasty and natural way to guard against a number of life-threatening conditions.

FURTHER READINGS

Dawson, Daniel. "USDA Predicts Global Olive Oil Production to Decrease Again." *Olive Oil Times*, June 5, 2020. Accessed Oct. 13, 2020. https://www.oliveoiltimes.com/world/usda-predicts-global-olive-oil-production-to-decrease-again/82721

"FDA Completes Review of Qualified Health Claim Petition for Oleic Acid and the Risk of Coronary Heart Disease." U.S. Food and Drug Administration, Nov. 19, 2018. Accessed Oct. 14, 2020. https://www.fda.gov/food/cfsan-constituent-updates/fda-completes-review-qualified-health-claim-petition-oleic-acid-and-risk-coronary-heart-disease

"Hunter Study Shows That Certain Olive Oils Kill Cancer Cells." Hunter College, Aug. 16, 2019. Accessed Oct. 14, 2020. https://hunter.cuny.edu/news/hunter-study-shows-that-certain-olive-oils-kill-cancer-cells/

Lopez, Sergio, et al. "Chapter 154–Oleic Acid: The Main Component of Olive Oil in Postprandial Metabolic Processes." *Olives and Olive Oil in Health and Disease Prevention*, Preedy, Victor R. and Watson, Ronald Ross, eds. London, England: Academic Press, Elsevier, 2010, p. 1385–1393.

Menendez, J.A., et al. "Oleic Acid, the Main Monounsaturated Fatty Acid of Olive Oil, Suppresses Her-2/neu (erbB-2) Expression and Synergistically Enhances the Growth Inhibitory Effects of Trastuzumab (Herception) in Breast Cancer Cells with Her-2/neu

Oncogene Amplification." *Annals of Oncology*, Mar. 2005, 16(3), 359–371. Accessed Oct. 13, 2020. https://pubmed.ncbi.nlm.nih.gov/15642702/
"Olive Oil." U.S. Department of Agriculture, Apr. 1, 2020. Accessed Oct. 13, 2020. https://ndb.nal.usda.gov/fdc-app.html#/food-details/789038/nutrients
Rueda-Clausen, Christian F., et al. "Olive, Soybean and Palm Oils Intake Have a Similar Acute Detrimental Effect Over the Endothelial Function in Healthy Young Subjects." *Nutrition, Metabolism, and Cardiovascular Diseases*, Jan. 2007, 17(1), 50–57. Accessed Oct. 14, 2020. https://pubmed.ncbi.nlm.nih.gov/17174226/
Schwingshackl, Lukas; Christoph, Marina; and Hoffmann, Georg. "Effects of Olive Oil on Markers of Inflammation and Endothelial Function—A Systematic Review and Meta-analysis." *Nutrients*, Sept. 2015, 7(9), 7651–7675. Accessed Oct. 14, 2020. https://www.ncbi.nlm.nih.gov/pmc/articles/PMC4586551/
Shahbandeh, M. "U.S. Olive Oil Consumption 2000–2019." Statista, Jan. 30, 2020. Accessed Oct. 13, 2020. https://www.statista.com/statistics/288368/olive-oil-consumption-united-states/
Terés, S., et al. "Oleic Acid Content Is Responsible for the Reduction in Blood Pressure Induced by Olive Oil." *Proceedings of the National Academy of Sciences United States of America*, Sept. 16, 2008, 105(37), 13811–13816. Accessed Oct. 14, 2020.
Vogel, R.A. "Brachial Artery Ultrasound: A Noninvasive Tool in the Assessment of Triglyceride-Rich Lipoproteins." *Clinical Cardiology*, June 1999, 22(6 Suppl), 1134–1139. Accessed Oct. 14, 2020. https://pubmed.ncbi.nlm.nih.gov/10376195/
Vogel, R.A., et al. "The Postprandial Effect of Components of the Mediterranean Diet on Endothelial Function." *Journal of the American College of Cardiology*, Nov. 1, 2000, 36(5), 1455–1460. Accessed Oct. 14, 2020. https://pubmed.ncbi.nlm.nih.gov/11079642/

Organic Foods

WHAT ARE THEY?

Organic foods are grown and processed according to USDA guidelines for use of natural substances and farming methods. Produce can be labeled organic if it comes from seed that has not been genetically modified and if it grows in soil that has not had any prohibited substance, such as synthetic fertilizers or pesticides, applied to it for the previous three years. Some synthetic substances have been approved by the USDA for use in organic farming, because of their low impact on the environment or on human health.

Organic meat and poultry must come from animals raised in living conditions that are suitable for their natural behavior, that is, free-ranging cattle and fowl. Animals must be fed on 100 percent organic feed or they must be allowed to forage in pastures that have not been treated with synthetic pesticides, herbicides, or fertilizers.

Processed foods labeled organic, including dairy products, fruit and vegetable juices, preserves, and baked goods, must be made with ingredients that were produced in fields, orchards, vineyards, and so on that follow organic guidelines. Yogurts and cheese may contain nonagricultural ingredients like enzymes to stimulate the culture, but they must come from dairy cattle (or plant sources) raised in organic conditions. Baking soda, yeast, vitamins, and dairy cultures are all permitted, but they must not be genetically modified.

Products with labels that say "Made with organic [ingredient]" contain at least 70 percent organically produced ingredients; the rest may be synthetic or otherwise, but they cannot be genetically modified or created with any of the USDA's "excluded methods" for organic labeling, including "a variety of methods to genetically modify organisms or influence their growth and development by means that are not possible under natural conditions or processes," including "cell fusion, microencapsulation and macroencapsulation, and recombinant DNA technology (including gene deletion, gene doubling, introducing a foreign gene, and changing the positions of genes when achieved by recombinant DNA technology)."

To qualify for organic labeling, farms must keep an organic systems plan that documents the practices and the step-by-step procedures employed to comply with the USDA's requirements.

CURRENT CONSUMPTION STATISTICS AND TRENDS

Sales of organic foods and products reached $55.1 billion in the United States in 2019, a 5 percent increase over 2018. In the first quarter of 2020, the pantry stocking phenomenon that seized the country at the beginning of the COVID-19 pandemic drove organic food sales up by more than 50 percent. The trend continued into the spring with a 20 percent jump in sales over the previous year, particularly organic milk and eggs. Even packaged and frozen organic prepared foods saw double-digit increases as people cooked at home for almost every meal.

The 2020 Organic Industry Survey, released in June 2020, noted that produce drove the increase in organic food sales in 2019, with sales up to $18 billion, nearly 5 percent over the previous year. The market for these foods turns out to be millennials and younger buyers, the generations that grew up with organic foods in their parents' refrigerators. Dairy grew at a slower rate of 2 percent over 2018, while meat, poultry, and fish make up the smallest category of organic food sales at just $1.4 billion—though this represents 10 percent growth over 2018. A significant segment of this is held by poultry, which accounted for $865 million in sales in 2019. Organic condiments—ketchup, sauces, mustard, and the like—and spices remain smaller markets, but they too saw growth in 2019.

NUTRITIONAL INFORMATION

No sweeping generalization can or should be made about whether all organic foods are healthier or more nutritious than conventionally grown and processed foods.

Some studies indicate that some organic produce may have an increased level of nutrients over conventional produce, particularly in flavonoids (antioxidants). Feeding livestock on natural feedstock instead of processed feed does generate higher levels of omega-3 fatty acids in meat, eggs, and dairy products (see Grass-Fed Beef earlier in this book).

More to the point, the reduction in synthetic pesticide residue, as well as the drop in levels of toxic metals often found in conventionally grown crops, means that organic foods transfer far less of these substances to the human body. "The difference in health outcomes is unclear because of safety regulations for maximum levels of residue allowed on conventional products," according to the Mayo Clinic's information on organic foods and nutrition.

HISTORY

Organic farming is not a new concept; agrarian societies practiced farming without chemicals for thousands of years before the Industrial Revolution and advances in biochemistry produced affordable, effective, synthetic fertilizers and pesticides. The use of these chemical solutions increased farm production dramatically, especially as large, gas-powered farm machinery allowed farmers to cultivate bigger fields. With increased human populations in big cities as people left farms behind to work in factories, corporate farms began to overtake the nation's agricultural sector, producing enough food to feed people who no longer grew their own.

In the early 1900s, Sir Albert Howard, a British botanist, and his wife, Gabrielle, moved to Pusa, Bengal, India, where they learned and documented the traditional farming practices used there. Howard wrote the 1940 book *An Agricultural Testament*, in which he and his wife detailed what they had seen and why these practices were superior to the farming that had become the norm in the Western world. In the same year, another British nobleman, Walter James, also known as Lord Northbourne, saw publication of his book *Look to the Land*, in which he imagined an approach to farming that emphasized balance and natural methods. Others around the world came to the same conclusions around the same time: Lady Eve Balfour, whose book *The Living Soil* detailed her own four-year experiment with "nonintensive" farming; and Masanobu Fukuoka, a Japanese microbiologist who left his profession to work on his family's farm and developed his own method of "natural farming."

With the coming of World War II, innovations in farming to feed the troops came fast and furious, including methods for irrigating huge fields and more automated farm machines. Accompanying these advancements were new pesticides including DDT, which soon turned out to be one of the most toxic and dangerous chemicals in a farmer's arsenal.

After the war and the subsequent population explosion, world leaders began to expect food shortages that would result in worldwide starvation if farmers did not produce even more abundant crops and bigger harvests. Not everyone saw this trend and believed that new, modern farming methods were the answer, however:

American farmer J.I. Rodale and others turned to what Rodale termed "organic gardening," a return to raising food without synthetic chemicals and aggressive mechanization.

Then came the book that changed the course of pesticide development: *Silent Spring*, Rachel Carson's stunning 1962 treatise on the harmful effects of DDT and a range of other pesticides, their effects on the environment at large, and on animals and humans. The book launched the modern ecology movement and played a key role in getting the U.S. government to ban the use of DDT, saving many bird species from extinction including the bald eagle and the peregrine falcon.

The organic farming movement was off and growing, keeping pace with environmental causes through the 1970s. Rodale founded Rodale Press, through which he distributed information about the impact of nonorganic farming methods and best practices in organic agriculture to date. The movement struggled in the 1980s even as it grew, because different farmers and organizations disagreed on what "organic" actually meant and what was and was not acceptable practice. This changed in 1990 with the Organic Foods Production Act, which established nationwide standards for organic food and fiber production, placing the USDA in charge of regulating the industry. The USDA worked with farmers to develop rules and finally published them in 2002.

THE CONTROVERSY

Organic produce and meat come at a higher price point in supermarkets and often at farm markets as well—so many consumers wonder if eating "clean" foods grown and raised without synthetic pesticides, antibiotics, or GMOs actually provides more food value than their conventionally raised counterparts.

There is no simple answer to this. Comparative analysis of organically and conventionally grown produce shows a modestly higher level of phenolic compounds in organic fruit and vegetables, antioxidants that may help guard against cancer—but conventionally grown produce has these compounds as well.

Most organic produce also has less pesticide residue on it than produce grown using synthetic pesticides, although sprayed pesticides from neighboring farms can blow onto organic produce and remain there until the fruit or vegetables are washed in a consumer's home. Organic farms use pesticides as well, though these come from natural sources. Any produce consumers purchase probably has some residue of natural or synthetic chemicals and should be washed before using or eating.

Dairy products from organically raised cattle and grass-fed meats have been found to be higher in ALA, an omega-3 fatty acid, than grain-fed meat. ALA may lower the risk of cardiovascular disease and slow down cancer cells' growth rate, making it a valuable part of a healthy diet. (See Grass-Fed Beef for more discussion of this.)

What organic foods do *not* contain is high levels of antibiotics, and this may be one of their most important advantages. While animals raised on organic farms may receive some antibiotics, the levels are far lower than those in animals raised on conventional dairy and poultry farms, making them a lesser contributor to antimicrobial resistance in consumers. Antibiotics in the foods we eat transfer to our bodies, allowing bacteria to build a tolerance to their use. When someone has an infection and needs an antibiotic, they may find that the germs in their system have already built up so much tolerance to the medication that the antibiotic the doctor prescribes does not work. Eating organic meats and dairy products can help consumers avoid this potentially dangerous situation.

Numerous studies have examined whether organic foods are healthier than conventional foods, as Mie et al. (2017) discovered in a comprehensive literature review of the human health implications of organic foods. Mie concluded that eating organic foods may reduce the risk of allergies and may have a positive impact for people trying to maintain a healthy weight. Some studies indicated that certain pesticides have a negative impact on children's cognitive development, but details on which pesticides do this have yet to be researched thoroughly.

One of the clear benefits of organic foods is the significantly lower levels of cadmium found in them, particularly in cereal grains and leafy vegetables. Cadmium, a toxic heavy metal, may get into the soil in agricultural areas where mining and smelting take place nearby. It travels through the air and comes to rest on plowed ground in farm fields, and some crops are particularly adept at pulling the metal out of the soil and into their own tissue. (This being said, most people who have high levels of cadmium in their bodies invite it in by smoking cigarettes, which can contain significant amounts of it.) Too much cadmium can cause kidney issues that may lead to kidney failure. It is also a carcinogen, placing the consumer at increased risk of lung, endometrium, bladder, and breast cancer. While whole grains and vegetables may provide a way for cadmium to enter the body, these foods and other high-fiber choices are also the best way to carry it back out. Eating organic foods can lower the risk of accumulating this metal, as studies have shown that organically grown grains and produce have lower levels of cadmium.

Overall, however, "I think people believe these food are better for them, but we really don't know that they are," said Kathy McManus, registered dietician and director of the Department of Nutrition at Brigham and Women's Hospital, an affiliate of Harvard University. "There've been a number of studies examining the macro- and micronutrient content, but whether organically or conventionally grown, the foods are really similar for vitamins, minerals, and carbohydrates." She concluded, "At this time, after examining the data, I don't see any nutritional reasons to choose organic foods over conventional."

In other words, the benefits have more to do with individual choice and concerns than with nutrition or scientific fact. Organic foods have their advantages; whether these are worth the additional cost is entirely up to the consumer.

FURTHER READINGS

Greger, Michael. "How to Reduce Your Dietary Cadmium Absorption." NitritionFacts.org, Oct. 15, 2015. Accessed Oct. 14, 2020. https://nutritionfacts.org/2015/10/15/how-to-reduce-your-dietary-cadmium-absorption/

"History of Organic Farming in the U.S." Sustainable Agriculture Research and Education. Accessed Oct. 14, 2020. https://www.sare.org/publications/transitioning-to-organic-production/history-of-organic-farming-in-the-united-states/

Kim, Kijoon, et al. "Dietary Cadmium Intake and Sources in the US." *Nutrients*, Jan. 2019, 11(1), 2. Accessed Oct. 14, 2020. https://www.ncbi.nlm.nih.gov/pmc/articles/PMC6356330/

Mayo Clinic staff. "Organic Foods: Are They Safer? More Nutritious?" Mayo Clinic, Apr. 8, 2020. Accessed Oct. 14, 2020. https://www.mayoclinic.org/healthy-lifestyle/nutrition-and-healthy-eating/in-depth/organic-food/art-20043880

McEvoy, Miles. "Organic 101: What Organic Farming (and Processing) Doesn't Allow." U.S. Department of Agriculture, Feb. 21, 2017. Accessed Oct. 14, 2020. https://www.usda.gov/media/blog/2011/12/16/organic-101-what-organic-farming-and-processing-doesnt-allow

McNeil, Maggie. "COVID-19 Will Shape Organic Industry in 2020 After Banner Year in 2019." Organic Trade Association, June 9, 2020. Accessed Oct. 14, 2020. https://ota.com/news/press-releases/21328

Mie, Axel, et al. "Human Health Implications of Organic Food and Organic Agriculture: A Comprehensive Review." *Environmental Health*, 2017, 16, 111. Accessed Oct. 14, 2020. https://www.ncbi.nlm.nih.gov/pmc/articles/PMC5658984/

"Should You Go Organic?" Harvard Health Publishing, Harvard Medical School, Sept. 2015. Accessed Oct. 14, 2020. https://www.health.harvard.edu/staying-healthy/should-you-go-organic

Phosphorus-Containing Food Additives

WHAT ARE THEY?

Some preservatives added to packaged and ready-to-eat foods contain phosphorus, a mineral required by the body to work with calcium to build healthy bones and teeth. Dicalcium phosphate, disodium phosphate, monosodium phosphate, phosphoric acid, sodium hexameta-phosphate, trisodium phosphate, sodium tripolyphosphate, and tetrasodium pyrophosphate (TSPP) are all names of preservatives, emulsifiers, and stabilizers that contain phosphorus as a major ingredient. Phosphorus helps extend the shelf life of packaged products including meats, cheeses, baked goods, chocolate, and some beverages, while enhancing flavor, aiding in leavening and yeast stimulation, and conditioning and stabilizing dough for baked goods. These wide-ranging attributes have made it an additive of choice for an increasing array of products. Phosphoric acid also sharpens the flavors of carbonated soft drinks; in particular, it gives cola its satisfying acidity.

Phosphates serve as emulsifiers for dairy products including yogurt, milk and milk-based beverages, pudding, ice cream, cheesecake, and processed cheeses.

CURRENT CONSUMPTION STATISTICS AND TRENDS

The market for phosphorus used in food additives topped $1.4 billion in the United States in 2015 and is expected to continue to grow significantly through 2024. Meat and seafood processing represents the largest share of this market, with sales above $150 million in 2015, followed by dairy, beverages, and bakery products. The meat, fish, and poultry markets prefer phosphate-based preservatives because the alkaline nature of phosphate helps to maintain the pH balance in these products. Sales of canned meats and fish were already forecasted for major growth to keep pace with consumers' busy lifestyles, but the pantry-stocking behavior of the 2020 pandemic pushed these sales even higher than expected.

NUTRITIONAL INFORMATION

Phosphorus helps the body repair its own cells and tissue and makes protein our bodies need to grow. It assists in kidney function, movement of muscles, maintaining a regular heartbeat, and communication between nerves.

HISTORY

Since Hennig Brand's discovery of phosphorus in urine in 1669, the glow-in-the-dark element revealed itself in ground-up bones and then in bird and bat guano, making it a substance that could be harvested from massive bird colonies on guano-covered islands, if someone determined that there could be value in such a distasteful enterprise. The reason to do so emerged in a groundbreaking book published in 1840: chemist Justin Von Liebig's *Organic Chemistry and Its Application to Agriculture and Physiology*, in which he provided a suggested method for mixing mineral phosphate with sulfuric acid to create a solution that could be used as a nutrient-rich fertilizer. John Bennet Lawes, an English agricultural scientist, patented a fertilizer in 1842 that he made using Von Liebig's guidelines and essentially launched the manmade fertilizer industry.

Mining operations began in the 1840s and soon depleted the guano islands of the mineral, just as less noxious methods of acquiring phosphorus from sedimentary phosphate rock started to take hold. Phosphorus mining continues today, with most of the world's supply coming from mines in Morocco, China, Algeria, and Syria.

Other chemists, particularly those in the food industry, soon began to explore the ways that phosphorus could be combined with other elements to produce additives that benefitted packaged goods. Disodium phosphate, for example, prevents condensed milk from coagulating, and it keeps instant pudding mix from caking while encouraging it to thicken when mixed with milk; it also makes instant cream of wheat cook faster. Heating this compound turns it into TSPP, which makes marshmallows hold together and preserves imitation crab, canned tuna, and meat alternatives like soy-based "meats." TSPP is applied to dental floss and used in toothpaste to repel calcium and magnesium in saliva, thus fighting tartar buildup between teeth.

THE CONTROVERSY

Excess phosphorus usually leaves the body through urine, but too much phosphorus can be harmful. An excess of this mineral can weaken bones by pulling calcium out of them and depositing the calcium in other places, including blood vessels, the heart, lungs, or eyes. These tiny deposits can build up over time, causing a heart attack or stroke or even death.

A study by Qunibi (2004) found that 12 percent of patients in stage 5 chronic kidney disease (CKD) died of hyperphosphatemia, an elevated serum phosphate concentration. High phosphorus levels have long been known to be a danger for kidney disease patients, but the extent of the threat has turned out to be higher than understood. Early in the 2010s, researchers also discovered a correlation between high-normal serum phosphate levels and cardiovascular events (heart attack and stroke), increasing our understanding of the impact phosphate additives in food may have on overall health.

"Inorganic phosphate in food additives is effectively absorbed and can measurably elevate the serum phosphate concentration in patients with advanced CKD," said Eberhard Ritz et al. in a paper published in a German journal in 2012. People who eat more processed and fast food can have vascular damage and calcification that can lead to serious illness, they concluded: "The public should be informed that added phosphate is damaging to health."

For healthy people who eat fresh food rather than processed meals and who maintain an active lifestyle, there is less danger of adverse effect. People who make packaged products staples in their diet, and whose lives are more sedentary, could find their phosphorus levels artificially elevated by inorganic phosphorus. Kidney disease sufferers are most at risk, because compromised kidneys struggle to process and expel phosphorus their bodies collect from food. A normal level of phosphorus is 2.5–4.5 mg/dL, but it can rise quickly for someone who eats a lot of packaged baked goods, fast food, cola, flavored waters, ready-to-eat or frozen meals, deli meats, snacks like tortilla chips, corn chips, and cheese puffs; and processed cheeses.

Patients with advanced kidney disease or kidney failure follow a strict diet that dramatically reduces the amount of organic phosphorus they take in, minimizing or eliminating foods in which it occurs naturally, like cheese and other dairy products, nuts, beans, organ meats, shellfish, and whole grains. Processed foods may add inorganic phosphorus to the load without them realizing that they are taking in more than their kidneys can handle.

The FDA requires that all preservatives be identified on food labeling, along with a statement of their purpose—for example, you may see a statement like this in the ingredients: "Sodium phosphate to preserve freshness." This indicates to consumers that phosphorus is an ingredient, but not how much of their RDA (currently 700 mg) they will consume in a serving. Nephrologists and researchers are working to bring the risks of phosphorus intake to the attention of the FDA, to convince this governing body to require a listing of the amount of phosphorus on the Nutrition Facts panel. If they succeed in making this listing mandatory, it will likely raise awareness among consumers of the need to monitor their daily phosphorus intake as one more step in taking control of their own good health and avoiding the chronic diseases and conditions that can result from too much phosphorus in their diet.

In addition, the 2006 Framingham Osteoporosis Study linked phosphoric acid in sugared cola drinks to reduced bone mineral density (BMD) in women, which in turn leads to osteoporosis. The study used a food frequency questionnaire to collect information from more than 2,500 people on a wide range of variables including body mass, height, age, energy intake, physical activity, smoking, consumption of alcohol, calcium, vitamin D, and caffeine intake aside from cola, as well as menopausal status in women; the researchers then used dual-energy X-ray absorptiometry (DEXA) scans to measure BMD. Women who drank full-sugar cola daily had significantly lower BMD at each of their hips (though not at the spine), and the results were nearly the same for diet cola. The researchers concluded that the combination of phosphoric acid and caffeine adversely affects bone density in women, although it does not do the same in men.

With these health issues in mind and in an effort to draw conclusions about the use of phosphorus as a food additive, researcher Allison Cooke conducted an extensive review of 110 primary research articles in 2017, in an effort to identify substantial evidence that dietary phosphorus or phosphates do (or do not) cause health issues in human beings. "The lack of conclusive evidence prevented the drawing of firm conclusions about the safety and possible risks of food-additive phosphate in the general population," she summed up her work, "which is consonant with the overall assessments of authoritative institutions who have concluded that available data are insufficient to make the required determinations."

In 2018, however, a twelve-week experiment conducted with mice as part of the Dallas Heart Study determined that administering high amounts of phosphates to the mice reduced the time they spent in moderate to vigorous physical exercise and increased the amount of time they spent doing nothing. The phosphates did not change the mice's body weight or heart function, but it reduced their uptake of oxygen, their spontaneous activity, and use of their treadmill and led to "downregulation of genes involved in fatty acid synthesis, release, and oxidation." They concluded that too much phosphate in their diet had a detrimental effect on muscle metabolism and capacity for exercise, independent of any direct effect on heart muscle. "Dietary [phosphates] may represent a novel and modifiable target to reduce physical inactivity associated with the Western diet," their report closed. Before the food industry begins to move away from versatile phosphates, however, this hypothesis would need to be proved conclusively in human subjects.

The FDA continues to include additives containing phosphorus on its GRAS list, generally regarding them as safe for human consumption. Until conclusively proven otherwise, these substances remain in foods and may provide a nutritional element to some, while posing a potential health hazard to others.

FURTHER READINGS

Ahuja, Kunal, et al. "Food Phosphate Market Size by Product . . ." Global Market Insights, Apr. 2017. Accessed Oct. 15, 2020. https://www.gminsights.com/industry-analysis/food-phosphate-market

Borgi, Lea. "Inclusion of Phosphorus in the Nutrition Facts Label." *Clinical Journal of the American Society of Nephrology*, Jan. 2019, 14(1) 139–140. Accessed Oct. 15, 2020. https://cjasn.asnjournals.org/content/14/1/139

Cooke, Allison. "Dietary Food-Additive Phosphate and Human Health Outcomes." *Comprehensive Reviews in Food Science and Food Safety*, Wiley Online Library, Aug. 1, 2017. Accessed Oct. 15, 2020. https://onlinelibrary.wiley.com/doi/full/10.1111/1541-4337.12275

"Phosphorus and Your Diet." National Kidney Foundation, Apr. 18, 2019. Accessed Oct. 15, 2020. https://www.kidney.org/atoz/content/phosphorus

Poghni, Peri-Okonny, et al. "High Phosphate Diet Induces Exercise Intolerance and Impairs Fatty Acid Metabolism in Mice." *Circulation*, Jan. 7, 2019, 139, 1422–1434. Accessed Oct. 15, 2020. https://www.ahajournals.org/doi/10.1161/CIRCULATIONAHA.118.037550

Qunibi, Wajeh Y. "Consequences of Hyperphosphatemia in Patients with End Stage Renal Disease." *Kidney International*, 2004, 66(90), S8–S12. Accessed Oct. 26, 2020. https://www.kidney-international.org/article/S0085-2538(15)50371-2/pdf

Ritz, Eberhard, et al. "Phosphate Additives in Food—A Health Risk." *Deutsches Arzteblatt International*, Jan. 2012, 109(4), 49–55. Accessed Oct. 15, 2020. https://www.ncbi.nlm.nih.gov/pmc/articles/PMC3278747/

Slack, A.V. "Phosphoric Acid, Part 1." New York: Marcel Dekker Inc, 1968. Located at "Phosphoric Acid History," ML2R Consultancy. Accessed Oct. 15, 2020. http://ml2r consultancy.com/phosphoric-acid-history/

Tucker, Katherine, et al. "Colas, But Not Other Carbonated Beverages, Are Associated with Low Bone Mineral Density in Older Women: The Framingham Osteoporosis Study." *American Journal of Clinical Nutrition*, Oct. 2006, 84(4), 936–942. Accessed Oct. 15, 2020. https://academic.oup.com/ajcn/article/84/4/936/4632980

Uribanni, Jaime. "Phosphorus Homeostatis in Normal Health and in Chronic Kidney Disease Patients with Special Emphasis on Dietary Phosphorus Intake." *Seminars in Dialysis*, July—Aug. 2007, 20(4), 295–301. Accessed Oct. 15, 2020. https://pubmed.ncbi.nlm.nih.gov/17635818/

Plant-Based Meats

WHAT ARE THEY?

Relatively new nonmeat products that taste like meat, including brand names like the Impossible™ Burger and Beyond Meat™, have the appearance, mouth-feel, and taste of ground beef—but they contain no animal-based products. These products are made from plant-based materials and other ingredients and they are cholesterol-free, making them an attractive alternative to beef.

CURRENT CONSUMPTION STATISTICS AND TRENDS

Plant-based burgers have been marketed directly to meat eaters rather than to vegetarians or vegans and they have scored in a big way. *NBC News* reported in late 2019 that up to 90 percent of the consumers of these burgers, "chicken" wings, and meatballs are omnivores, choosing the meatless alternative for its perceived healthful benefits. Since their nationwide introduction in 2017, sales of Impossible Foods' plant-based meat alternatives have grown from $118.7 million in their first year to $192.1 million in 2019. Nearly 80 percent of this growth comes directly from the availability of the Impossible Burger at Burger King and Beyond Meat products at Carl's Jr., Del Taco, A&W, and other fast-food restaurants. Both companies' products are also available in grocery stores including Target and Wal-Mart, among many others.

NUTRITIONAL INFORMATION

A 4-ounce serving of an Impossible burger contains 19 g of protein from plant-based sources, 14 g of fat, of which 8 g is saturated fat; 370 mg of sodium, and 9 g of carbohydrates, including 3 g of dietary fiber. The burger contains less than 1 g of sugar. Its vitamin content includes 2,350 percent of the RDA of thiamin, 130 percent of the RDA of vitamin B_{12}, and significant percentages of iron, potassium, riboflavin, niacin, folate, phosphorus, and zinc.

A four-ounce serving of Beyond Meat's burger contains 20 g of protein, 18 g of fat, of which 5 g is saturated fat; no cholesterol, 350 mg of sodium, and 5 g of carbohydrates, including 2 g of fiber. It provides 20 percent of the RDA of iron, as well as some calcium.

The Impossible burger's ingredients include soy protein concentrate, coconut oil, sunflower oil, and small amounts (less than 2 percent) of potato protein, methylcellulose, yeast extract, dextrose, food starch modified, soy leghemoglobin (more on this later), salt, antioxidants, soy protein isolate, and added vitamins and minerals.

Beyond Meat's burger contains pea protein, canola oil, coconut oil, rice protein, natural flavors, cocoa butter, mung bean protein, methylcellulose, potato starch, apple extract, pomegranate extract, salt, potassium chloride, vinegar, lemon juice concentrate, sunflower lecithin, and beet juice extract.

HISTORY

Beyond Meat introduced its first products to the vegan and vegetarian markets in 2012, but these early entries did not mimic the taste, appearance, and texture of actual meat. That breakthrough came to market in 2016, when founder Ethan Brown compiled an unorthodox research team of scientists with background in biochemistry, biophysics, plant science, technology, and chemistry to determine what made meat look and taste the way it does. The company moved into a former airport hangar in El Segundo, California, and turned its attention to recreating its product line to create a meat-eating experience that could begin to convince carnivores to choose plant-based products.

Brown's primary concern: livestock's impact on the environment, particularly in the massive amounts of methane that the dairy, beef, and hog industries expel into the air. Methane from livestock contributes between 6 and 7 percent of the total greenhouse gas emissions on earth. If people could get the same satisfaction they enjoy when eating a burger—one of the most popular foods in America—while eating something that tasted the same but did not come from a ruminating animal, demand for beef and pork might decrease. Fewer animals on smaller farms could have a positive effect on the planet's greenhouse gas load, which could benefit the environment. Cattle also require about 99 percent more water than, for example, potatoes do to produce a serving of food; raising fewer cattle could extend the planet's water supply dramatically.

Meanwhile, development of a new line of nonmeat products that look and taste like meat became the life's work of biochemist Patrick O. Brown (no relation to Ethan), a professor emeritus at Stanford University. His quest to discover what makes meat taste like meat began in 2009, when he took a temporary leave from Stanford to devote his time to the problem of moving the world's population away from animal meat.

Pat Brown worked with a team of scientists to understand the ingredients that make beef look, feel, and taste like beef. He landed on a plant-based substance called heme, a molecule found in all living things that distributes oxygen through the bloodstream or through the stems and leaves of a plant. Heme has the added benefit of giving meat its meaty taste. In particular, the team determined that soy leghemoglobin, found in the molecules of soy plants, can be fermented with yeast in a laboratory much the same way that beermakers use fermentation. This allowed them to generate large amounts of heme, making it possible to scale up their production of plant-based meat that tastes like beef.

Impossible Foods tested prototypes for nearly three years before unveiling its meatless burgers in the restaurants of four top chefs in 2016. The response led the company to begin scaling up production in 2017, and within a year, Impossible Burgers arrived in major fast-food chains, restaurants, and supermarkets across the country. With such a positive reception for its initial products, the company has turned its attention to other animal foods to duplicate the appearance, taste, and texture of pork, chicken, fish, and eggs with plant products.

THE CONTROVERSY

Any new food product generates curiosity and criticism; it may even draw a faction that believes that the unfamiliar substance that makes the product taste good also must be bad for us. Impossible Foods' use of a naturally occurring ingredient, soy leghemoglobin (heme), drew doubters, critics, and eventual opposition when it became clear that the company reproduced heme in a laboratory, using the common practice of fermentation with yeast to move its plant-based meat to mass production.

When Impossible Foods concluded its own testing of soy leghemoglobin using independent consultants, it approached the FDA in 2015 to receive its GRAS status for soy leghemoglobin. The FDA responded with concern that the fermented ingredient had never been consumed by humans, so the potential was there for it to emerge as an allergen for some people. A memo prepared for a phone discussion with company officials said that the FDA believed the documentation presented by Impossible Foods did not "establish the safety of soy leghemoglobin for consumption," nor did it "point to a general recognition of safety."

Impossible Foods did not require the FDA's full approval of its products—in fact, most new ingredients do not need their approval if the company producing them hires consultants to run tests and confirm the food's safety. The government agency did not conclude that soy leghemoglobin was actually unsafe; it stated it could not be sure that the ingredient did not pose a health hazard. Impossible Foods re-petitioned the FDA and finally received approval with their November 2018 petition that defined soy leghemoglobin as a color additive.

"The FDA reviewed the information and data submitted by the firm, as well as other relevant information, and concluded that there is a reasonable certainty of no harm from this use of soy leghemoglobin as a color additive," the FDA's statement said.

On the surface, it looked like the issue had been resolved. The rule allowed for a thirty-day comment period for objections, however, and the Center for Food Safety moved quickly to object. "Unfortunately, the Impossible Burger might just be too good to be true," the organization says on its website. "We believe that replacing conventional animal products with ultra-processed, poorly studied, and under regulated genetically engineered products is NOT the solution to our factory farm and climate crisis."

The CFS says that Impossible Foods used genetically modified (GMO) soybeans instead of organic ones. CFS mentions that it does not know for certain how Impossible Foods processes its soy; this is usually done with an alcohol solvent, which removes healthful isoflavones from the soy. The organization goes on to say that this GMO soy is usually sprayed with the herbicide glyphosate, a known carcinogen—but CFS does not know whether the soy used by Impossible Foods actually contains this herbicide.

Next, CFS objected to heme on the basis of it being a new product for consumers, citing the process of any food receiving the GRAS status as "a weak regulatory process . . . where the company does its own research and chooses its own reviewers to self-certify that its product is safe for human consumption."

When soy leghemoglobin received its GRAS rating from the FDA, the Center for Food Safety filed a lawsuit challenging the GRAS regulatory process as a "food additive loophole that the Impossible Burger went through, allowing it and many other novel food substances to unlawfully evade government analysis and approval before coming to market."

The feud between Impossible Foods and the Center for Food Safety continued to escalate throughout 2019, until the FDA reviewed the objections CFS submitted and determined that they "do not raise genuine and substantial issues of fact and do not provide any substantive evidence that would justify a hearing or otherwise provide a basis for revoking the amendment to the regulations." The rule approving soy leghemoglobin as safe became effective on December 17, 2019.

Impossible Foods also says on its website that in 2019, it removed the ingredients that contained gluten from its recipe and that its Impossible Burger 2.0 does not contain gluten. It does, however, contain the genetically engineered ingredients soy leghemoglobin and soy protein.

> To make heme: We take the DNA for soy leghemoglobin, insert it into yeast, and ferment the yeast. By making our heme using genetic engineering, we avoid growing and digging up soy plants to harvest heme (from the root nodules), which would promote erosion and release carbon stored in the soil. The method we've adopted enables us to produce heme sustainably at high volume and make meat from plants for millions of people that is delicious, nutritious and vastly more sustainable than meat from animals. We also source genetically engineered soy protein from farms in Iowa, Minnesota and Illinois that meet the highest standards for health, safety, and sustainability.

For the record, Beyond Meat makes a point of distancing itself from its competitor's controversy by saying outright on its website, "Our ingredients are simple and made from plants—without GMOs or synthetically produced ingredients."

Whether consumers see Impossible Foods' use of a genetically engineered ingredient as a deal-breaker or a competitive advantage, sales of both Impossible's and Beyond's burgers have created a new market niche that will be fascinating to watch as they produce new products and, perhaps, make a dent in the beef market.

FURTHER READINGS

Brown, Pat. "The Mission That Motivates Us." Impossible Foods, Jan. 23, 2018. Accessed Oct. 16, 2020. https://medium.com/impossible-foods/the-mission-that-motivates-us-d4d7de61665

"Carbon, Methane Emissions and the Dairy Cow." Penn State Extension, May 5, 2016. Accessed Oct. 16, 2020. https://extension.psu.edu/carbon-methane-emissions-and-the-dairy-cow
Clinton, Patrick. "The Impossible Burger Is Probably Safe. So Why Is Everyone Worked Up About 'Heme'?" *The Counter*, Aug. 22, 2017. Accessed Oct. 16, 2020. https://thecounter.org/plant-blood-soy-leghemoglobin-impossible-burger/
Hanson, Jaydee. "Our Beef with the GMO Impossible Burger." Center for Food Safety, June 20, 2019. Accessed Oct. 16, 2020. https://www.centerforfoodsafety.org/blog/5628/our-beef-with-the-gmo-impossible-burger
Lee, Joey. "5 Myths Impossible Burger Is Serving Up." Center for Food Safety, Oct. 28, 2019. Accessed Oct. 16, 2020. https://www.centerforfoodsafety.org/blog/5783/5-myths-impossible-burger-is-serving-up
"Original Constituent Update: FDA Authorizes Soy Leghemoglobin as a Color Additive." U.S. Food and Drug Administration, July 31, 2019. Accessed Oct. 16, 2020. https://www.fda.gov/food/cfsan-constituent-updates/fda-announces-effective-date-final-rule-adding-soy-leghemoglobin-list-color-additives-exempt
Strom, Stephanie. "Impossible Burger's 'Secret Sauce' Highlights Challenges of Food Tech." *New York Times*, Aug. 8, 2017. Accessed Oct. 16, 2020. https://www.nytimes.com/2017/08/08/business/impossible-burger-food-meat.html
"What Are the Ingredients?" Impossible Foods. Accessed Oct. 26, 2020. https://faq.impossiblefoods.com/hc/en-us/articles/360018937494-What-are-the-ingredients-
"What Is Beyond Meat Made Out Of?" and "Beyond Burger." Beyond Meat website. Accessed Oct. 26, 2020. https://www.beyondmeat.com/products/the-beyond-burger/

Probiotics

WHAT ARE THEY?

Probiotics are live bacteria or yeasts that the body needs and that already live in people's bodies. These beneficial bacteria help the body maintain a balance between good and bad bacteria, so the good bacteria can eliminate the overabundance of bad bacteria caused by infection or illness. These good microbes live in the gut, urinary tract, vagina, mouth, and lungs, and on skin.

CURRENT CONSUMPTION STATISTICS AND TRENDS

The U.S. probiotics market, including foods and supplements, reached $49.4 billion in 2018 and is expected to increase to $69.3 billion by 2023. Probiotic-fortified foods and their perceived health benefits drive this continued growth. Specific yeasts, including a tropical yeast known as *Saccharomyces boulardii*, play a role in this growth as research concludes that they have a positive effect on human health. Around the world, probiotic yogurts have found a market in

China, Brazil, India, and Japan, and drinks and even candies containing probiotics have become more available in these countries.

NUTRITIONAL INFORMATION

Probiotic supplements or foods containing these good bacteria may help the body deal with certain medical conditions involving the digestive system, urinary tract, gums, vagina, upper respiratory tract, and skin. Foods that contain probiotics include yogurt, buttermilk, kombucha, kefir, sourdough bread, cottage cheese, tempeh, kimchi, miso soup, and pickles.

HISTORY

"Death sits in the bowels," wrote Hippocrates two millennia ago, and anyone with irritable bowel syndrome, inflammatory bowel disease, or a number of other gut-based conditions would most likely agree. The search for a simple solution for digestive discomfort began thousands of years ago and has had many stopgap remedies, but the first real understanding of the role good bacteria may play in the process came in the early 1900s, when Louis Pasteur found the bacteria responsible for fermentation. This discovery became the jumping-off point for Ilya Ilych "Elie" Mechnikov, a Russian scientist who later won the Nobel Prize for his work linking fermented dairy products with the remarkable longevity of rural residents in Bulgaria, many of whom lived to be well over 100 years old. Metchnikoff made the connection between the elder Bulgarians and a bacterium, *Bulgarian bacillus*, discovered by young physician Stamen Grigorov, and suggested that the secret to their long lives might lie in the consumption of these bacilli in their "soured milk" or yogurt.

"The dependence of the intestinal microbes on the food makes it possible to adopt measures to modify the flora in our bodies and to replace the harmful microbes by useful microbes," he postulated. This fitting description of the function of probiotics became the first major step in moving the science forward.

In the 1990s, the science of gastroenterology made its next major leap with research into the gut microbiome, a concerted effort to understand the microbes in the digestive tract. This led to the World Health Organization's formal definition of probiotics in 2001, which in turn encouraged researchers to apply even more effort to comprehend how these good bacteria worked within the human body. Definitions of microbial strains emerged quickly, as did the realization that some probiotics die in stomach acid and never get the opportunity to do their job. From this greater knowledge came the probiotics industry, with products to help these bacteria survive the trip into the intestines, and the identification of specific probiotics contained in various products so consumers could learn which ones they needed and wanted.

THE CONTROVERSY

Many products containing probiotics have proclamations of "digestive health" or "gut wellness" on their packaging, but not all containers of yogurt or kombucha drinks deliver the same good bacteria to the digestive system—and the claim that a product contains probiotics does not guarantee healthful benefits.

Probiotics make their way to consumers as dietary supplements, food ingredients, and drugs. Dietary supplements do not require FDA approval to come to market, although they are regulated to some extent: Supplement manufacturers cannot make health claims on their packaging (such as "Cures Irritable Bowel Syndrome") without proving the effectiveness of their product to the FDA. If the product does indeed have the curative property it claims, it may be reclassified as a drug and it then must meet stricter FDA requirements for pharmaceuticals—including proof that the drug can be used by human beings safely.

A wide and far-reaching range of studies have been conducted on probiotics to fully understand their role in the gut microbiome and their potential for promoting good health. Some studies have found that they prevent the diarrhea that comes with taking antibiotics, especially the loose stools caused by the bacterium *Clostridium difficile*. This, however, seems to be true only in young to middle-aged people; elderly people do not benefit, according to a review of thirty studies conducted in 2016—although of the more than 7,000 participants in the studies, only a few people older than sixty-five years were included, so the difference in effectiveness could be circumstantial rather than statistical. In another group of studies, children appeared to benefit from the use of probiotics while they were on antibiotics, with no harmful effects.

Studies of the effects of probiotics on constipation have not generated conclusive results to date, though they have shown evidence that adults receive some benefits, while children generally do not. Still more studies have been inconclusive at best on whether patients with diarrhea caused by cancer treatment, diverticular disease, or Crohn's disease get better when using probiotics. A 2014 review of twenty-one studies of 1,700 patients with ulcerative colitis did find that adding probiotics to their treatment could help them maintain remission. The same was true of a 2018 review of fifty-three studies of patients with irritable bowel syndrome, although the researchers could not determine which specific probiotic bacteria or combinations may have produced the positive effects.

Despite the sheer quantity of studies on this topic, very few solid conclusions have come of them. The variety of probiotic bacteria to study and the difficulty in isolating one probiotic for a specific study has slowed progress, so that scientists have considerable work left to do to determine which bacteria affect which issues. The question of dosage also remains open: How much yogurt or kefir a person should consume to generate a positive effect on their bowel issues has yet to be determined. Some people seem to benefit from including probiotics in their diets, while others do not—and researchers struggle to pinpoint the reasons for this.

One thing that researchers do seem to agree on is that probiotics are largely safe; the only harmful effects documented tend to be in people who have severe illnesses or who are fighting autoimmune diseases. High-risk patients should discuss adding probiotics to their therapy with the physicians in charge of their care, to be sure that the benefits will outweigh the potential harm. In particular, research indicates that people who are immunocompromised should avoid probiotics, as they may cause infection or production of harmful substances in the digestive tract.

FURTHER READINGS

Gasbarrini, Giovanni, et al. "Probiotics History." *Clinical Gastroenterology*, Nov./Dec. 2016, 50, 5116–5119. Accessed Oct. 16, 2020. https://journals.lww.com/jcge/fulltext/2016/11001/probiotics_history.3.aspx

Lamb, Stephen. "A Brief History of Probiotics." ZBiotics, July 4, 2019. Accessed Oct. 16, 2020. https://zbiotics.com/blogs/journal/a-brief-history-of-probiotics-span-a-walk-down-memory-lane-from-the-beginning-of-probiotic-history-to-today-and-beyond-span

"Probiotics." Cleveland Clinic, Mar. 9, 2020. Accessed Oct. 16, 2020. https://my.clevelandclinic.org/health/articles/14598-probiotics

"Probiotics: What You Need To Know." National Center for Complementary and Integrative Health, Aug. 2019. Accessed Oct. 16, 2020. https://www.nccih.nih.gov/health/probiotics-what-you-need-to-know

"Probiotics Market by Application . . . Global Forecast to 2023." Markets and Markets. Accessed Oct. 16, 2020. https://www.marketsandmarkets.com/Market-Reports/probiotic-market-advanced-technologies-and-global-market-69.html

Raw Milk

WHAT IS IT?

Raw milk is milk that has not been pasteurized to kill potentially harmful bacteria like *Brucella*, *Campylobacter*, *Cryptosporidium*, *Escherichia coli*, *Listeria monocytogenes*, and *Salmonella*, which can be present in milk from cows, goats, or any other animal. These germs can cause food poisoning, with symptoms including persistent diarrhea, stomach cramps, vomiting, and diseases that can lead to paralysis or even death.

The Raw Milk Institute publishes standards that today's raw milk farmers are expected to follow. These include frequent testing for coliform bacteria and standard plate count; testing for pathogens including *Campylobacter*, *Listeria monocytogenes*, and *Salmonella*; and ensuring that the cattle are free of tuberculosis and brucellosis. These farms also commit to using processes for milk handling and management that prevent bacteria from entering the milk supply and to selling milk that is only from their own farm, eliminating the concern that milk from other farms may not be produced using the same standards.

CURRENT CONSUMPTION STATISTICS AND TRENDS

Only about 3.2 percent of the U.S. population drinks raw milk, and only 1.6 percent eats cheese made from raw milk. A report in the June 2017 issue of the journal *Emerging Infectious Diseases* determined that raw milk drinkers are 840 times more likely to contract a foodborne illness than people who drink pasteurized milk, and they are forty-five times more likely to be hospitalized if they get sick.

Outbreaks of illness associated with dairy consumption cause 760 illnesses per year on average, representing 96 percent of illnesses caused by contaminated dairy products. "As consumption of unpasteurized dairy products grows, illnesses will increase steadily; a doubling in the consumption of unpasteurized milk or cheese could increase outbreak-related illnesses by 96%," wrote researchers Solenne Costard et al. in their 2017 report to the Centers for Disease Control.

NUTRITIONAL INFORMATION

Raw milk contains much the same nutrients as pasteurized milk; these nutrients—calcium, iodine, phosphorus, potassium, protein, and vitamins B_2 and B_{12}—are not affected by the pasteurization process. Pasteurizing milk does render some enzymes in milk inactive, but these enzymes are not required by humans for good health. There is no additional nutritional benefit to drinking raw milk instead of pasteurized milk.

Proponents of raw milk argue that unpasteurized milk provides immunity-building properties that strengthen the gut microbiome and help humans resist diseases.

HISTORY

As the Industrial Revolution took hold and people moved from farms into cities to work in all kinds of manufacturing jobs, families had to abandon the common practice of keeping their own dairy cows. Apartment buildings and congested conditions in crowded cities did not allow for livestock, so families bought milk at the local market—and the origins of this milk could be something of a mystery.

The facts became a sobering piece of food history: Milk production facilities kept cattle confined to stalls where they were fed the remains of grains fermented in nearby beer and whisky factories. Noxious and devoid of nutrition, this mash in turn led to cows producing milk that crossed the line into unpalatability. Worse, the conditions in which cows produced this milk led to rampant spread of disease-causing bacteria, and the delivery of this milk to consumers—often in open pails that could contain all manner of contaminants—only maximized the spread of germs throughout cities. Children drank most of this milk, encouraged to do so by their unsuspecting parents who believed milk to be a most healthful food . . . and children got sick, and many of them died. In 1882, when scientist Robert Koch discovered the bacterium that causes tuberculosis, it became possible to trace the source of this disease throughout the late 1800s—and much of it spread through contaminated milk.

The public outcry pushed reform of milk production to the top of activists' lists in the late nineteenth century—right about when Louis Pasteur developed his method for destroying germs using heat. Pasteur's interest focused on wine and beer, but the process translated perfectly to milk, and by 1920, states began to require pasteurization of milk by law.

It took time to introduce pasteurization into every dairy operation in the country, but the process worked. In 1938, 25 percent of all disease outbreaks from contaminated food and water came from milk; by 2005, milk was responsible for just 1 percent of such outbreaks, and most of these were from raw milk.

The federal government worked with the dairy industry to make pasteurization a standard, but it did not ban outright the sale of raw milk. Some states took the initiative and banned raw milk sales on their own, but some did not; some cities and counties passed their own laws against it, but its sale still continued in rural areas. From 1973 to 1992, forty-six outbreaks of disease from drinking raw milk took place throughout the country, and forty of them were in states where raw milk was legal.

The FDA began its work to eliminate raw milk from the nation in 1973, a process that made its way through the courts until it finally became a regulation in 1987, banning the shipping of raw milk across state lines and mandating the pasteurization of all milk and dairy products in final packaged form. This did not end the sale of raw milk in some states, however, and from 1998 to 2005, disease outbreaks traced to raw milk were blamed in 1007 illnesses, 104 hospitalizations, and 2 deaths.

As soon as the regulation locked into place, however, people who advocate for raw milk began to find one another and form organizations. Today the raw milk industry accounts for a tiny percentage of the milk-buying population, and consumers in thirty states can purchase this milk in stores or directly from dairy farms that follow strict procedures for raising their cattle in healthy, sanitary conditions. This care of the animals and the process has not eliminated the potential for harm that pasteurization renders moot, but it allows people who want raw milk to feel somewhat more confident about consuming it than they could in the late nineteenth century.

THE CONTROVERSY

The FDA bans the interstate sale or distribution of raw milk at the federal level, requiring that all milk and other dairy products sold across state lines be pasteurized. States can determine what happens to milk produced within their own boundaries, however, and as of 2016, thirteen states permit the sale of raw milk in grocery stores or any other retail establishments. Seventeen other states permit farms to sell raw milk directly to consumers, but it cannot be sold in stores. Eight states allow consumers to acquire raw milk through "cow-share" agreements, that is, two neighboring families raising livestock and sharing milk from their own cows. In the remaining twenty states, all sale of raw milk is prohibited; however, drinking raw milk is legal in all fifty states.

Why do people want to drink raw milk, a potentially contaminated and dangerous food, when so much evidence points to the healthful benefits of pasteurized milk? Mullin and Belkoff (2014) conducted an online survey of raw milk consumers to attempt to get to the bottom of this issue. They discovered that the primary reason respondents gave for their use of raw milk was that they believed it was healthier than pasteurized milk. The Raw Milk Institute, an organization dedicated to ensuring that raw milk is "clean and safe," details some of these health benefits on its website, linking to a list of studies cited by the British Columbia Herdshare Association. Some of these studies suggest that infants and children below the age of six who drank "farm milk," or unpasteurized milk, are less likely to develop hay fever, asthma, and an overall tendency toward allergies in their first few years of life. Some studies that ask adults to recall what they were fed early in life also connect a lack of asthma or allergies with childhood consumption of milk directly from farms.

About 30 percent of the respondents to Mullin and Belkoff's survey said that they had some stomach or intestinal discomfort from drinking pasteurized milk, which disappeared when they drank raw milk. Some proponents of raw milk believe that lactose intolerance comes as a direct result of the pasteurization process, which they say eliminates the catalyst with which the body produces the lactase enzyme that makes lactose digestible. According to information provided by the Raw Milk Institute, people who first began drinking milk from animals many millennia ago did not have the lactase persistence gene that produced the lactase enzyme. Drinking raw milk allowed them to develop this gene and digest milk without issues, according to the institute; lactose intolerance, then, became a problem caused by pasteurization.

Despite the standards set by the Raw Milk Institute for farmers who sell raw milk, the Centers for Disease Control warn of the potential for contamination of the milk on these farms. Animal feces coming into direct contact with the milk may spread bacteria that is not detected by testing the animals. Bacteria can live on cattle's skin and find its way into the milk, and processing equipment may not be cleaned as regularly as a sanitary process requires. Insects, rodents, and other carriers of bacteria and germs can get into the milk. Dairy workers who do not follow sanitation procedures to the letter may bring dirty clothing, shoes, or hands in contact with milk. Pasteurization kills all of these bacteria that raw milk allows to remain.

"Negative tests do not guarantee that raw milk is safe to drink," the CDC says. "Milk that is safe one day may not be safe the next day. Also, tests do not always detect low levels of contamination. People have become very sick from drinking raw milk that came from farms that regularly tested their milk for bacteria and whose owners were sure that their milk was safe." Labeling the raw milk "organic" is not a promise of purity either, as organic practices do not screen out bacteria. If organic milk is important to consumers, they can buy pasteurized organic milk at any supermarket.

Like so many medical controversies, some research bears out one side, while some supports the other. Consumers make their own decisions about what is best for their tables and their families, so the question remains: Is consumption of raw milk worth the risk of diseases caused by the bacteria that may or may not be found in the milk? Or is drinking pasteurized milk, which can be guaranteed not to contain these bacteria, the better option? The FDA and the CDC see pasteurization as a clear choice; the final decision is up to you.

FURTHER READINGS

Beach, Coral. "What Are the Odds? 840 Times More Likely for Raw Milk Drinkers." *Food Safety News*, May 2, 2017. Accessed Oct. 18, 2020. https://www.foodsafetynews.com/2017/05/what-are-the-odds-840-times-more-likely-for-raw-milk-drinkers/

"Common Standards." Raw Milk Institute. Accessed Oct. 18, 2020. https://static1.squarespace.com/static/5c930aceaf4683e69e2cd577/t/5f6c9d780f04ca43911015ca/1600953721374/2020+RAWMI+Common+Standards+Final.pdf

Costard, Solenne, et al. "Outbreak-Related Disease Burden Associated with Consumption of Unpasteurized Cow's Milk and Cheese, United States 2009–2014." *Emerging Infectious Diseases*, Center for Disease Control and Prevention, June 2017, 23(6). Accessed Oct. 18, 2020. https://wwwnc.cdc.gov/eid/article/23/6/15-1603_article

Marler, Bill. "A Legal History of Raw Milk in the United States." Marler Clark, Dec. 31, 2007. Accessed Oct. 18, 2020. https://www.marlerblog.com/lawyer-oped/a-legal-history-of-raw-milk-in-the-united-states/

McAfee, Mark; and Smith, Sarah. "Why Humans Drink (RAW) Milk." Raw Milk Institute, July 7, 2020. Accessed Oct. 18, 2020. https://www.rawmilkinstitute.org/updates/why-humans-drink-raw-milk

Mullin, Gerard; and Belkoff, Stephen. "Survey to Determine Why People Drink Raw Milk." *Global Advances in Health and Medicine*, Nov. 2014, 3(6), 19–24. Accessed Oct. 18, 2020. https://www.ncbi.nlm.nih.gov/pmc/articles/PMC4268642/

"Raw Milk Laws State-by-State." Britannica ProCon.org, Apr. 19, 2016. Accessed Oct. 18, 2020. https://milk.procon.org/raw-milk-laws-state-by-state/

"Raw Milk Questions and Answers." Centers for Disease Control and Prevention. Accessed Oct. 18, 2020. https://www.cdc.gov/foodsafety/rawmilk/raw-milk-questions-and-answers.html

"The Health Benefits of Raw Milk." British Columbia Herdshare Association. Accessed Oct. 18, 2020. http://bcherdshare.org/the-health-benefits-of-raw-milk/
"The History of Raw Milk and Pasteurization." Food (Policy) For Thought, May 6, 2014. Accessed Oct. 18, 2020. http://foodpolicyforthought.com/2014/05/06/the-history-of-raw-milk-and-pasteurization/

Red Meat

WHAT IS IT?

Science defines red meat as any meat that contains high levels of myoglobin, a protein that binds iron and oxygen. Myoglobin is found in all mammals, but in higher concentrations in cattle, sheep, and hogs, and it contains hemes, which give meat its red color. According to the USDA, red meat includes beef, pork, veal, and lamb; game meats including venison, bison, and hare are also red meats.

CURRENT CONSUMPTION STATISTICS AND TRENDS

Beef production reached 27.2 billion pounds in 2019, an increase of 1.1 percent over 2018. Pork production came in just behind beef at 27.1 billion pounds, a 2.9 percent increase over the year before. Per capita annual consumption of beef fell slightly in 2019 to 56.8 pounds per person, while pork increased to fifty-one pounds per person. Veal production reached 74 million pounds in 2019, dropping steadily from 143 million pounds in 2008, with most of this consumed in restaurants; households consume less than half a pound of veal annually. Lamb, once favored by households, has dropped to about 1 pound per person annually over the last several years.

NUTRITIONAL INFORMATION

Red meat provides protein, a critically important factor in maintaining strong bones and muscles. Beef and pork also include all of the amino acids the body requires to grow and maintain good health.

A serving of beef may contain as much as 20 percent saturated and monosaturated fat, though many cuts are leaner. Some of this fat comes in the form of CLA, which plays a role in controlling body weight.

Beef and pork contain many vitamins and minerals including high amounts of iron, as well as vitamins B_6 and B_{12}, zinc, selenium, niacin, and phosphorus. They also provide creatine, which delivers energy to muscles; taurine for heart and muscle function; and the antioxidant glutathione. Both meats contain cholesterol, but this form of dietary cholesterol does not affect levels in the blood. Pork also provides thiamine, a B vitamin essential to several body functions.

HISTORY

Indigenous people in North America hunted game animals for meat since the first nomads set foot on this continent, many of them following the migrations of large mammals across the Great Plains and through the forests. Meat became a staple on the American table when the first European settlers landed on the continent's eastern shores. The forests and plains provided abundant sources of meat for the taking, with deer, rabbit, and a wide range of other animals readily available. As settlers moved west, they found herds of bison, elk, and deer, so the need to raise domestic livestock did not come about until these herds had been hunted to depletion. Cattle, pigs, sheep, and goats imported from Europe and the United Kingdom began to provide the meat Americans needed to feed their families over the course of the nineteenth century, according to Roger Horowitz's seminal 2006 book *Putting Meat on the American Table*.

In 1800, 90 percent of Americans lived on farms and raised their own food and livestock. Horowitz derived per capita meat consumption estimates from livestock production in the 1830s and determined that people ate about 178 pounds of meat per year, though not all of this was red meat.

As industry took hold and thousands of people left their farms to seek their fortune in cities, the need to centralize farming of domestic animals became clear to Congress, and laws began to codify the processes of animal husbandry and large-scale farming. The Homestead Act of 1862 spurred on the development of family farms and the Morrill Act made it possible to set aside land for agricultural colleges to study crop management and animal husbandry, among many other subjects. These two laws smoothed the road to the growth of farming in the Midwest and beyond, creating larger farms where thousands of head of livestock could be produced annually.

Once cattle arrived from the ranches, meat had to be packaged for sale, so meat-packing plants sprang up in major cities across the country. Stockyards in Chicago, Philadelphia, Cincinnati, Kansas City, and Omaha took in live cattle right off the railroad cars and processed it for markets, loading it back onto trains for transport to cities and communities throughout the country. The growth of this industry soon necessitated the passage of laws about product quality, ensuring that only fresh, healthful meat reached consumers' tables. The Meat Inspection Act of 1906 forced the issue, eliminating meat not fit for consumption from the supply chain.

And not a moment too soon. Horowitz discovered a survey conducted in 1909 that found that poorer households ate about 136 pounds of meat annually, while wealthier families ate more than 200 pounds of beef, veal, pork, lamb, sausage, and poultry. Families in the survey spent three times as much money on beef as they did on pork, although households in the southern states demonstrated a preference for pork, enough so that it became known as the "staff of life" in Georgia, appearing on the table with every meal.

As refrigeration arrived in households in the twentieth century, the need to cure meats for preservation became less important. Salt pork, once a staple in southern homes, all but disappeared from tables in white households, as families chose bacon or ham instead. Black families, often working with less income than whites, still chose salt pork and the cheapest cuts to maintain their consumption of meats. In the Great Depression of the 1930s, meat consumption dropped precipitously in virtually all homes, with even the most prosperous families eating 132 pounds per year instead of their accustomed 200. This rebounded after World War II, with beef and poultry topping the list of favorites and beef coming out on top. In the 1960s, people ate more meat, especially beef, than they ever had before: Rural families ate 50 percent more beef than pork, and urban families devoured 205.2 pounds of meat annually, with more than half of it beef.

With this desire for beef and pork came methods for expanding production and farms that could raise tens of thousands of cattle at once. The most widespread method for factory farming involves keeping the cattle confined in stalls for the last six to nine months of their lives, during which they are "finished" on a diet of fortified grain to increase their size quickly. This makes farm-raised cattle different from the free-range animals hunted by our ancestors—those animals of early America roamed through the woods and fields and fed on grasses, making them generally leaner than farm-raised cattle. Today's beef and pork come from animals that lead sedentary lives and eat processed grains, making their meat fattier than the meat eaten in the 1700s and 1800s. (See Grass-Fed Beef earlier in the book for more information on this.)

In 1955, nutritional scientist Ancel Keys at the University of Minnesota called for large-scale clinical studies on the connection between diet and health. By this time, researchers had discovered the effects of cholesterol in blood vessels and its direct link to heart attack and stroke. Why some people's cholesterol levels were much higher than others remained unknown, so Keys and others embarked on major clinical studies to determine if what people ate had any relationship to their heart health. Keys found a definite link between dietary cholesterol and heart disease, as did the famous Framingham Heart Study, and before the decade ended, several other laboratories had determined that eliminating dietary saturated fats and replacing them with unsaturated fats could reduce blood cholesterol significantly. Red meat, both processed and unprocessed, landed on the list of foods to limit or avoid entirely.

Beginning in the 1950s and still part of its advice today, the American Heart Association recommends avoiding red meat because of its saturated fat and cholesterol content and eating chicken, fish, and beans as the proteins of choice to keep cholesterol levels under control and avoid heart disease.

THE CONTROVERSY

It seemed like decided science: Red meat's saturated fat and cholesterol make it a less than optimal choice for a healthy diet, even in moderation. This became common wisdom more than seventy years ago, although it does not seem to have reduced consumption of red meat, as beef continues to be the most popular source of protein in the American diet. The American Heart Association, American Cancer Society, American Diabetes Association, and the National Kidney Foundation all recommend limiting or eliminating red meat.

Studies spanning decades have shown a consistent correlation between red meat consumption and increased serum cholesterol, and a number of studies have also linked red meat with the body's potential for developing cancer, especially colon cancer. All of this got flipped on its ear, however, by a set of five studies published in October 2019 by an international team of researchers who examined the effects of red meat and processed meat on a range of health issues, including heart disease, cancer, diabetes, and dying young.

The five studies, published in *Annals of Internal Medicine*, conducted meta-analyses of existing research and came to the same conclusions:

> Low to very-low-certainty evidence that diets lower in red meat compared with those higher in red meat have minimal or no influence on all-cause mortality, cancer mortality, cardiovascular mortality, myocardial infarction [heart attack], stroke, diabetes, and incidence of gastrointestinal and gynecologic cancer. Our results highlight the uncertainty regarding causal relationships between red meat consumption and major cardiometabolic and cancer outcomes.

This led to an explosion of headlines in newspapers and on websites around the world, proclaiming that there was "no need to cut down red and processed meat for health reasons," as a headline in *Science News* announced.

Bradley Johnston, corresponding author on the reviews and an associate professor at McMaster University, where the reviews took place, told *Science Daily*, "This is not just another study on red and processed meat, but a series of high quality systematic reviews resulting in recommendations we think are far more transparent, robust and reliable."

The scientific community, however, didn't buy it. "This new red meat and processed meat recommendation was based on flawed methodology and a misinterpretation of nutritional evidence," said Frank Hu, MD, chair of the Department of Nutrition at Harvard University's T.H. Chan School of Public Health. "The authors used a method often applied to randomized clinical trials for drugs and devices, which is typically not feasible in nutritional studies." He cited evidence accumulated over decades that link a steady diet of red and processed meat with higher risk for heart disease, cancer, and diabetes.

The pivot point for these studies, however, is the amount of red and processed meat required to increase the disease risk. "The evidence shows that people with a relatively low intake have lower health risks," Hu said in an article about the studies on the Harvard Health Publishing website. "A general recommendation is that people should stick to no more than two to three servings per week."

One thing that all researchers seem to agree about is the difference between red meat and processed meat—bacon, sausage, cured meats like corned beef and pastrami, and other delicatessen meats. Processed meats contain chemicals and additives that strengthen the link to diseases, Hu noted. "Again, there is not a specific amount that is considered safe, so you should keep processed meat intake to a minimum," he said.

FURTHER READINGS

Arnason, Atii. "Beef 101: Nutrition Facts and Health Effects." Healthline, Apr. 4, 2019. Accessed Oct. 18, 2020. https://www.healthline.com/nutrition/foods/beef

Arnason, Atii. "Pork 101: Nutrition Facts and Health Effects." Healthline, Mar. 28, 2019. Accessed Oct. 18, 2020. https://www.healthline.com/nutrition/foods/pork

Bray, Robert W. "History of Meat Science." American Meat Science Association, 1997. Accessed Oct. 19, 2020. https://meatscience.org/about-amsa/history-mission/history-of-meat-science

Garbarino, Jeanne. "Cholesterol and Controversy: Past, Present and Future." *Scientific American*, Nov. 15, 2011. Accessed Oct. 19, 2020. https://blogs.scientificamerican.com/guest-blog/cholesterol-confusion-and-why-we-should-rethink-our-approach-to-statin-therapy/

Gunnars, Kris. "Is Red Meat Bad for You, or Good? An Objective Look." Healthline, May 22, 2018. Accessed Oct. 19, 2020. https://www.healthline.com/nutrition/is-red-meat-bad-for-you-or-good

Horowitz, Roger. "Putting Meat on the American Table: Taste, Technology, Transformation." Baltimore, MD: Johns Hopkins University Press, 2006.

"Meat, Poultry, and Fish: Picking Healthy Proteins." American Heart Association. Accessed Oct. 19, 2020. https://www.heart.org/en/healthy-living/healthy-eating/eat-smart/nutrition-basics/meat-poultry-and-fish-picking-healthy-proteins

Peel, Derrell. "2019 Meat Production and Consumption." Drovers, Apr. 4, 2019. Accessed Oct. 18, 2020. https://www.drovers.com/article/2019-meat-production-and-consumption

Teicholz, Nina. "How Americans Got Red Meat Wrong." *The Atlantic*, June 2, 2014. Accessed Oct. 19, 2020. https://www.theatlantic.com/health/archive/2014/06/how-americans-used-to-eat/371895/

Wein, Harrison. "Risk in Red Meat?" National Institutes of Health, Mar. 26, 2012. Accessed Oct. 19, 2020. https://www.nih.gov/news-events/nih-research-matters/risk-red-meat

"What's the Beef with Red Meat?" Harvard Health Publishing, Harvard Medical School, Feb. 2020. Accessed Oct. 19, 2020. https://www.health.harvard.edu/staying-healthy/whats-the-beef-with-red-meat

Zeraatkar, Dena, et al. "Effect of Lower Versus Higher Red Meat Intake on Cardiometabolic and Cancer Outcomes." *Annals of Internal Medicine*, Oct. 1, 2019. Accessed Oct. 19, 2020. https://www.acpjournals.org/doi/10.7326/M19-0622

Salt

WHAT IS IT?

The mineral compound sodium chloride (NaCl) can be found on every table around the world, obtained primarily through salt mining or desalination of seawater. As a nutrient, it is required for life in humans and animals.

CURRENT CONSUMPTION STATISTICS AND TRENDS

Americans consume about 3,400 mg of salt per day, or about 1½ teaspoons, well above the RDA of 2,300 mg (1 teaspoon). Children and teenagers may be taking in much more salt, especially if they eat packaged or processed foods, frozen dinners, or fast food on a regular basis. These foods contain much more salt than fresh foods do, even after unprocessed foods are cooked in a home kitchen.

NUTRITIONAL INFORMATION

Salt is a nutrient in itself, required by the human body to generate nerve impulses and to maintain the balance of fluids and electrolytes—the substances that produce electrical impulses between nerves to enable nerves and muscles to function. Salt keeps the body from dehydrating by retaining fluids. Humans need between 115 and 500 mg of salt per day to maintain optimal levels and more if they are in active situations that promote perspiration, such as playing a sport or manual labor. Most people consume much more salt than this: The FDA recommends that consumers reduce their daily salt intake to 2,300 mg or roughly one teaspoon per day.

HISTORY

It is impossible to say exactly when salt came into common usage, but its ever-present position as a seasoning for food came well before the beginning of recorded history. In 2700 BC, a Chinese treatise detailed more than forty different kinds of salt and described two methods for collecting them that do not stray far from today's modern mining practices. Salt served as currency in a number of ancient cultures and its use in trading made it particularly desirable and useful to early governments. Roman soldiers received salt in payment for their services ("salarium," the word for this, led to our current word "salary"). The Old Testament of the Judeo-Christian Bible talks about salt and coined the phrase "salt of the earth," a reference to purity of nature.

When Europeans arrived on the shores of what became North America, they found Native Americans harvesting salt on the island of St Maarten. Onondaga tribesmen in what would become New York State made salt by boiling the water of salt springs as a brine and taught this valuable process to colonialists. By 1800, the new Americans had established large salt production operations, especially in Kanawha, West Virginia, and began drilling for more brine in underwater salt springs.

Spanish and Portuguese fishermen reaching the shores of Newfoundland used the local salt to preserve their fish, as did French and English fleets as they arrived in the New World. Throughout the American Revolution and as explorers and settlers moved west, the availability of salt became an important question, and salt makers were vital to new settlements and expeditions. The Erie Canal allowed barges to ship New York State's mined salt, much of it from upstate and western New York, to the Great Lakes for transport to new settlements and burgeoning cities in the west. Even in the Civil War, the battle to capture Saltville, Virginia, for its salt processing plant became a critical goal for Union soldiers, who succeeded in taking possession of the town.

Drilling operations discovered underground salt deposits in New York, Ohio, Michigan, Kansas, Louisiana, Texas, and Utah, as well as in Canada in Ontario, New Brunswick, Quebec, and Nova Scotia, and conventional mining soon followed. Today salt is big business, keeping readily available a commodity no human can live without, used to bring out the flavor in food, to preserve foods by reducing their water content, leaving less for mold and other microbes to use; to give texture to bread dough and binding ability to processed meats; to prevent fermentation in making pickles, cheese, and sauerkraut; and to promote the development of color in processed meats and the golden color in bread crust. Just about every food we can name contains some salt, and a number of additives increase the sodium content, with names like sodium benzoate, sodium acetate, sodium ascorbate, sodium diacetate, and sodium nitrate or nitrite.

THE CONTROVERSY

The ubiquitous nature of salt, appearing in every packaged food and in so many processed meats and cheese, means that humans get a generous helping of salt with virtually every bite of food they consume. This means that our bodies take in much more salt than we need to sustain our good health. Whether or not this is a problem has been the subject of many studies, blurring the lines between healthy salt intake and the wages of excess sodium.

In 1904, a group of French doctors were the first to raise the red flag that there might be a connection between consumption of large amounts of salt and high blood pressure. Later, in a 1948 study by Kempner, 500 patients who had high blood pressure were treated with a diet containing 20 g of protein, a little fat, and less than half a gram of salt per day, as well as rice and fruit. The protein and rice diet improved blood pressure and even decreased the size of enlarged hearts, along with other benefits, but this bland diet did not catch on with the public despite its healthful effects. Throughout the next several decades, more researchers turned their attention to the question of salt and hypertension, running studies on rats, chimpanzees, and finally humans.

A famous study on disparate populations in Newfoundland provided some new insights: People in an inland county consumed between 6.7 and 7.3 g of salt per day as part of their regular diet, while a coastal community ate between 8.4 and 8.8 g of salt per day. About 15 percent of the inland community's population had high blood pressure, but many more of the coastal residents—27 percent—had elevated blood pressure, and the researchers concluded that their salt intake was the culprit. A similar study in the Solomon Islands produced the same kind of proof of salt's effect on hypertension.

INTERSALT, the largest study of its kind when it reached completion in 1988, used twenty-four-hour urinalysis to determine how much salt each of its 10,079 subjects aged twenty to fifty-nine consumed each day. The study found a direct correlation between salt intake and blood pressure, especially in older participants: Older people with higher salt intake had the highest blood pressure, while people of the same age with low salt consumption did not see an increase in blood pressure at all. The study indicated that blood pressure increases with age only if a person's salt intake is high. Equally important, lowering the sodium intake corrected the issue, decreasing systolic blood pressure.

Many more studies confirmed these findings and explored the issue further, but they all came to the same general conclusions: More salt correlated with higher blood pressure and lowering salt intake lowered blood pressure.

With as much as 29 percent of the world's population afflicted with high blood pressure, salt's role in causing hypertension continues to receive intensive study, despite most researchers considering the matter decided.

Why, then, is this long-held certainty of the link between salt and hypertension being called into question? Not every study lines up perfectly behind the effects of salt, most likely because salt is not the sole contributor to high blood pressure.

In April 2011, a meta-analysis of seven studies with a total of 6,250 participants found no direct correlation between reducing salt intake and lowering the risk of heart attack, stroke, or death. A study published in the *American Journal of Hypertension* in 2015 performed a cross-sectional analysis of 8,670 volunteers from the NutriNet-Santé study, a longitudinal web-based French study. Researchers used questionnaires to assess what participants ate, their blood pressure, and their lifestyle behaviors and concluded that age and body mass index are the main contributors to blood pressure issues. The study did not rule out the influence of salt—in fact, it did find that salt intake "was positively associated with [systolic blood pressure] in men but not in women." This study became one of the many quoted by the popular media, however, in disputing the effects of salt on raising blood pressure.

A study covered by *Medical News Today* in 2017, presented at that year's Experimental Biology conference, used participants in the Framingham Offspring Study to explore the effects of sodium on blood pressure over a period of sixteen years. The researchers found that participants who consumed less than 2,500 mg (2.5 g) of sodium daily had higher blood pressure than the people who ate foods with higher amounts of sodium. "While we expected dietary sodium intake to be positively associated with both [systolic blood pressure] and [diastolic blood pressure], the opposite was found," Moore et al. wrote. This study led some to conclude that both too much salt and too little salt can have an effect on blood pressure—a phenomenon that became known as the J curve—and in turn on a person's risk of developing heart disease.

None of these studies dismiss salt's influence on blood pressure entirely; they simply modify what earlier research revealed. What does skew the conclusions and their meaning are the headlines in the popular media: "High Blood Pressure: Sodium May Not Be the Culprit," when the study quoted says it is; "It's Time to End the War On Salt," quoting studies that do not suggest that salt consumption is a good thing; "A Spoonful of Salt Makes the Blood Pressure Go Down," when the article is about eliminating salt, not adding it.

In October 2020, Michael Jacobson, PhD, cofounder and former director of the Center for Science in the Public Interest (CSPI), published his book *Salt Wars: The Battle Over the Biggest Killer in the American Diet*. Jacobson has worked since 1977 to convince the federal government, particularly the FDA, to regulate salt the way it does sugar and fat. CSPI saw progress in the early 1980s when the FDA said it would work with the food manufacturing industry to lower sodium content in its foods, but the agency stopped short of actually regulating maximum salt levels, and the food industry continued to use salt as a flavor enhancer and preservative in many foods.

In 2010, the National Academy of Medicine recommended that the FDA set limits on sodium levels in food, but the FDA declined to act. Six years of pressure finally led the FDA to propose voluntary guidelines for sodium content, but when the new administration came into office at the beginning of 2017, salt and healthier eating were not its priorities. The effort stalled.

Jacobson discounts the findings of the 2017 study that suggest a J-curve in which a low-salt diet could be more harmful than a high-salt diet. "Researchers only looked at sodium intake on one day at the beginning of the study," he told *Medical News Today* in October 2020. "One day may not be representative of what a person is going to eat over the next five, ten, or twenty years." He also noted that most of the people in the study who ate foods low in sodium also had preexisting conditions like cancer or heart disease. "Those people may have intentionally lowered their sodium intake, so it wasn't that low sodium was causing disease, but that the disease was spurring people to consume less sodium."

CSPI struggles against another force that resists regulating salt: the food manufacturing industry's powerful lobbyists. "I think they fear that voluntary reductions would turn into mandatory restrictions," he said, with the potential for expensive changes in the way frozen and packaged foods are preserved. Sodium-based preservatives are very effective antimicrobials, because they reduce the water activity in foods, leaving little for microbes like mold to use for nourishment and growth. Finding another antimicrobial that is as effective and inexpensive as salt could prove difficult and costly.

There seems little doubt that salt raises blood pressure and causes health issues, even though a handful of studies have suggested otherwise. For the most current thinking, consumers should look to the most reliable sources: the extensive resources at the Centers for Disease Control and Prevention website, for example, which provide links to many studies as well as clear information about sodium and its effect on blood pressure.

FURTHER READINGS

Al-Zubaidi, Muhanad. "Salt and High Blood Pressure: Fact vs. Fiction." *Premier Health*, Mar. 5, 2020. Accessed Oct. 19, 2020. https://www.premierhealth.com/your-health/articles/women-wisdom-wellness-/salt-and-high-blood-pressure-fact-vs.-fiction

D'Ambrosio, Amanda. "Salt Slips From Regulatory Radar." *MedPage Today*, Oct. 20, 2020. Accessed Oct. 25, 2020. https://www.medpagetoday.com/primarycare/diet nutrition/89226

Feng, J. He, et al. "Does Reducing Salt Intake Increase Cardiovascular Mortality?" *Kidney International*, Oct. 1, 2011, 80(7), 696–698. Accessed Oct. 19, 2020. https://www.sciencedirect.com/science/article/pii/S0085253815551296

Ha, Sung Kyu. "Dietary Salt Intake and Hypertension." *Electrolytes and Blood Pressure*, June 2014, 12(1), 7–18. Accessed Oct. 19, 2020. https://www.ncbi.nlm.nih.gov/pmc/articles/PMC4105387/

"Heart Disease: Sodium." Centers for Disease Control and Prevention. Accessed Oct. 19, 2020. https://www.cdc.gov/heartdisease/sodium.htm

Jacobson, Michael F. *Salt Wars: The Battle Over the Biggest Killer in the American Diet*. Cambridge, MA: The MIT Press, Oct. 20, 2020.

Lelong, Helene, et al. "Relationship Between Nutrition and Blood Pressure: A Cross-Sectional Analysis From the NutriNet-Santé Study, a French Web-Based Cohort Study." *American Journal of Hypertension*, Mar. 2015, 28(3), 362–371. Accessed Oct. 19, 2020. https://academic.oup.com/ajh/article/28/3/362/2743418

Newman, Tim. "High Blood Pressure: Sodium May Not Be the Culprit." *Medical News Today*, Apr. 25, 2017. Accessed Oct. 19, 2020. https://www.medicalnewstoday.com/articles/317099

Wenner Moyer, Melinda. "It's Time to End the War on Salt." *Scientific American*, July 8, 2011. Accessed Oct. 19, 2020. https://www.scientificamerican.com/article/its-time-to-end-the-war-on-salt/

"You May Be Surprised by How Much Salt You're Eating." U.S. Food and Drug Administration, July 19, 2016. Accessed Oct. 19, 2020. https://www.fda.gov/consumers/consumer-updates/you-may-be-surprised-how-much-salt-youre-eating

Saturated Fat

WHAT IS IT?

Fats are made of two kinds of molecules: glycerol and fatty acids. They have long chains of carbon atoms that link to one another through single bonds (one point of contact) or double bonds (two points of contact). When the double bonds meet up with hydrogen, they form single bonds, breaking one of their bonds with another carbon atom to attach to the hydrogen atom. Saturated fats are completely saturated with hydrogen, with every carbon atom in their molecules linked with a hydrogen atom.

Saturated fats are solid at room temperature and include the fat that marbles red meats, the fat found under the skin of poultry, and the fat in cream, lard, butter, full-fat cheese, and whole milk. Plant fats tend to be unsaturated, although coconut oil is a saturated fat.

CURRENT CONSUMPTION STATISTICS AND TRENDS

The National Health and Nutrition Examination Survey for 2015–2020 determined that while federal recommendations limit saturated fat to less than 10 percent of total calories daily, people make foods that contain saturated fats an average of 11 percent of their daily intake, rising to as much as 12.6 percent for children. Only about 29 percent of Americans limit their saturated fats to 10 percent of their diet or less. The report notes that most of these saturated fats come from "mixed dishes," especially food choices that contain both meat and cheese: burgers, sandwiches, tacos, and pizza; as well as meat, poultry, and seafood dishes that features cheese; and rice, pasta, and grain dishes cooked with meat, cream, cheese, and/or butter. Snacks, desserts, and dairy products may also push the saturated fat content of a single meal past the 10 percent limit.

NUTRITIONAL INFORMATION

The FDA notes that saturated fat provides calories for energy, helps the body absorb some vitamins, and supports some functions, but the human body makes its own saturated fat, so it does not require any from food. Dietary guidelines from the FDA, the USDA, and other federal sources recommend that people make saturated fat less than 10 percent of their diet, replacing saturated fats with monounsaturated fat (such as olive oil) whenever possible.

HISTORY

People have eaten foods high in saturated fat since they felled their first mammoth thousands of years before recorded history, but our understanding of this kind of fat and its role in heart disease and other health issues did not come to the surface until the 1950s. Ancel Keys' Seven Countries study, in which he worked with researchers in Finland, Greece, Italy, Japan, the Netherlands, the United States, and Yugoslavia, discovered the association between saturated fat intake and heart disease mortality by examining 12,770 men aged forty to fifty-nine twice—once at the beginning of the study and once five years later. In the ensuing years, a number of the participants died of heart disease, and the study endeavored to link specific behaviors and body weight with this phenomenon. "Cigarette smoking, body fatness and relative bodyweight did not seem to explain population differences in incidence of the disorder, but there was a tendency for incidence to be related to the prevalence of hypertension, serum cholesterol values and saturated fatty acids in the diet," he wrote.

Researchers had observed the correlation between saturated fat consumption and cardiovascular issues, but the Framingham Heart Study, a groundbreaking long-term research effort, revealed the connection between high cholesterol and heart disease. How cholesterol became so high in some people remained a mystery, however, as men with cholesterol over 260 who had heart disease ate the same amount and kinds of fat as men whose cholesterol measured just 200.

Studies that involve participants remembering what they ate and how often they ate it are notoriously unreliable, as the subjects often don't recall what they consumed or they will give answers they believe the researchers want to hear, rather than admitting to an extra piece of cake or fast-food cheeseburger. This is what makes the Finnish Mental Hospital Trial a particularly interesting research effort: The crossover study of patients in two mental hospitals in Helsinki throughout the 1960s had the opportunity to control the diets of all of its participants. One hospital provided its patients with meals that featured butter and whole milk, while the other served food prepared with unsaturated vegetable oil and a substance called "filled milk," milk with the fat filtered out and replaced with vegetable oil. This continued for six years; then the two hospitals switched diets, and the process continued for another six years. The patients who had received the full-fat diet first saw their risk of dying from cardiovascular disease drop by 50 percent when they switched to the other diet—though most participants were not in the study for the entire twelve years, as patients came and went as their mental health declined or improved.

Studies throughout the 1970s clarified our understanding of cholesterol as a combination of LDL (bad) and HDL (good) particles, which led to further developments in dietary guidelines—including the realization that simply replacing saturated fat calories with carbohydrates reduces HDL cholesterol, an undesirable outcome, and increases triglycerides, which play a role in the development of metabolic syndrome and diabetes. Better guidelines were required, with an eye toward overall health rather than a specific focus on heart disease.

In 1977, the U.S. federal government codified its recommendations in a report, *Dietary Goals for the United States*, calling for reduced fat consumption, less salt, significantly reduced sugar, and a push to eat more fruits and vegetables, whole grains, poultry, and fish, and less high-fat foods including meats, eggs, and full-fat dairy products. This signaled the government's faith in the low-fat approach, though critics from the scientific community and from several food industries booed the recommendations, claiming that they were based on unproven theories about fat and sugar. Research continued to examine the fat question, however, and by the 1980s, enough studies pointed to the connection between saturated fat and heart disease that the medical community began to embrace the low-fat diet for patients who were overweight or who had signs and symptoms of heart disease.

The food industry got on board, but not in a way that promoted good health. What became known as the "Snackwell's phenomenon" centered on bringing products to market that could be touted as low fat, even though they still contained high levels of other ingredients that led to obesity. In particular, packaged foods like Snackwell's cookies replaced fat with sugar to create recipes that worked and cookies that tasted good, advertising them as a healthy choice. The campaign saw great success and such products filled grocery store shelves, but consuming them did nothing to aid in weight loss or improve people's health.

When the USDA released its food pyramid in 1992, underscoring the commitment to low-fat eating as the key to cardiovascular health, the American Heart Association began its heart-healthy seal of approval program, labeling low-fat foods as meeting the organization's criteria "for saturated fat and cholesterol for healthy people over age 2," even if these products were highly processed and loaded with sugar (e.g., Kellogg's Frosted Flakes and Pop Tarts qualified). Eliminating saturated fat became the primary goal for good health, no matter what else people ate. Studies throughout the 1990s and into the 2000s continued to find that reducing fat resulted in lower cholesterol, which in turn reduced the risk of heart disease.

Today our understanding of heart disease and its causes has broadened, and saturated fat remains one of the elements to avoid for better heart health as well as for the lower body weight that helps us avoid metabolic syndrome and diabetes. It is not the only cause of heart disease and other illnesses, however, and scientists still work to determine the one true diet for overall health.

Research has also shown that monounsaturated and polyunsaturated fats actually lower disease risk, news that returned vegetable oils, nuts, seeds, and fatty fish like salmon to the list of healthy choices. The removal of trans fats from many products and the ban of "partially hydrogenated" fat eliminated a well-documented enemy of human health from processed and fast foods. Saturated fats remain as the one fat researchers agree leads to obesity, heart disease, and other illnesses.

THE CONTROVERSY

With so much evidence that saturated fat contributes to a host of potentially deadly diseases, is it possible that this demon of unhealthy diets actually has some benefits? Or could it be that saturated fats are not the death blow to human health that science suggests they are?

The Atkins diet, introduced in the 1960s, gained sudden widespread popularity in the 2000s, taking the food industry in a low-carbohydrate direction. It focuses on replacing carbohydrates with, among other things, saturated fats like butter, cheese, high-fat meats, and coconut and palm oil. It pointed to studies whose results indicated that replacing saturated fat with carbohydrates increased the risk of heart attack and used these to draw the conclusion that saturated fats were a better choice than carbs. "The failure of low-fat dietary approaches is partially explained by the lack of understanding that when they lower their saturated fat intake, many people replace them with more carbohydrates. The culprit is not saturated fat per se," the Atkins website still stated in 2020. "If your carbohydrate intake is low, there's little reason to worry about saturated fat in your diet." This approach made low-carb dieters incorporate butter, cheese, and high-fat meats into their daily choices.

The ketogenic diet, introduced in the 1920s as a method for controlling epilepsy, rose to public consciousness in 1994 when it became the subject of an episode of NBC's *Dateline* and became very popular throughout the 2000s. Like Atkins, it promotes the replacement of almost all carbohydrates with high-fat meats, butter, cream, and cheese, as well as coconut oil, which is almost entirely saturated fat.

Both of these diets—and any other diet that reduces calorie intake—do lead to temporary weight loss, but their effect on heart health is largely unknown, and the small studies conducted to date provide conflicting results.

In 2014, *Annals of Internal Medicine* published a study (Chowdhury et al.) in which the researchers examined forty-nine observational studies involving more than 537,000 participants and twenty-seven randomized control trials with more than 105,000 participants, to attempt to eliminate study biases and determine if saturated fats truly are as harmful as the studies claimed. Their explosive conclusion: "Current evidence does not clearly support cardiovascular guidelines that encourage high consumption of polyunsaturated fatty acids and low consumption of total saturated fats."

This set off a firestorm of popular media stories proclaiming that "Butter is Back," further fueling a debate that continues to this day. A June 2020 discussion in the Great Debates in Nutrition section of the *American Journal of Clinical Nutrition* pitted Ronald Krauss, MD, of Children's Hospital Oakland Research Institute against Penny Kris-Etherton, PhD, of Pennsylvania State University on the topic of saturated fats and whether they should be reduced as much as possible in the human diet. Both experts placed the importance of a person's total diet over the significance of any single food or food group, and they agreed that saturated fats play a role in increasing LDL cholesterol. Whether or not limiting saturated fats actually reduces cholesterol and heart disease risk, however, turned out to be a question for debate. Krauss noted that evidence of this is inconclusive, even after decades of study. Kris-Etherton believed the evidence provides enough basis to recommend that people lower the amount of these fats they consume.

"To wait until all questions are answered before any recommendations are made to limit saturated fatty acids further ignores the evidence base we have which when implemented can prevent cardiovascular disease (and other diseases) in many people," Kris-Etherton said.

The one thing virtually all experts agree on, though, is that replacing saturated fats with simple carbohydrates like sugar, processed foods, and bread poses "substantial health risks," both Krauss and Kris-Etherton concluded.

So the debate continues. Until one randomized, double-blind, controlled study can provide a clear answer to the question, saturated fats remain a hotly contested issue, and ischemic heart disease remains the number one cause of death worldwide.

FURTHER READINGS

Chowdhury, Rajiv, et al. "Association of Dietary, Circulating, and Supplement Fatty Acids with Coronary Risk." *Annals of Internal Medicine*, Mar. 18, 2014. Accessed Oct. 20, 2020. https://www.acpjournals.org/doi/10.7326/M13-1788?articleid=1846638&atab=7

"Experts Debate Saturated Fat Consumption Guidelines for Americans." American Society of Nutrition, June 3, 2020. Accessed Oct. 20, 2020. https://medicalxpress.com/news/2020-06-experts-debate-saturated-fat-consumption.html

Forouhi, Nita G., et al. "Dietary Fat and Cardiometabolic Health: Evidence, Controversies, and Consensus for Guidance." *British Medical Journal*, 2018, 361: k2139. Accessed Oct. 20, 2020. https://www.ncbi.nlm.nih.gov/pmc/articles/PMC6053258/

Keys, A. "Coronary Heart Disease in Seven Countries." *Circulation*, 1970, 41(1), 186–195. Accessed Oct. 20, 2020. https://www.cabdirect.org/cabdirect/abstract/19711403775

Kritchevsky, David. "History of Recommendations to the Public About Dietary Fat." *Journal of Nutrition*, Feb. 1988, 128(2), 4495–4525. Accessed Oct. 20, 2020. https://academic.oup.com/jn/article/128/2/449S/4724049

LaBerge, Ann F. "How the Ideology of Low Fat Conquered America." *Journal of the History of Medicine and Allied Sciences*, Apr. 2008, 63(2), 139–177. Accessed Oct. 20, 2020. https://academic.oup.com/jhmas/article/63/2/139/772615

Miettinen, M., et al. "Effect of Cholesterol Lowering Diet on Mortality from Coronary Disease and Other Causes: A Twelve Year Trial in Men and Women." *Lancet*, Oct. 21, 1972, 2(7782), 835–838.

Soy

WHAT IS IT?

Soy is a protein that comes from the soybean, a legume native to East Asia and grown throughout the world. Many foods are made from soy, including tofu, soy milk, soy sauce, tempeh, edamame, natto, fermented bean paste, and textured vegetable protein (TVP). It is also one of the main protein sources in the feed of domestic animals bred for human consumption.

CURRENT CONSUMPTION STATISTICS AND TRENDS

The United States leads the world in raising soybeans, producing 3.5 billion bushels of soybeans in 2019 alone. This represented a significant decrease compared to 2018, however, when the nation produced 4.4 billion bushels, most of these in Illinois, Iowa, and Minnesota. The drop in production represents a corresponding reduction in demand for exports, caused by a decline in exports to China because of tariffs on U.S.-imported soybeans by the Chinese government. This tariff was imposed in response to tariffs on Chinese imports by the U.S. government.

NUTRITIONAL INFORMATION

Soybeans provide protein, dietary fiber, and nutrients including iron, manganese, phosphorus, folate, and several other B vitamins, vitamin K, magnesium, zinc, and potassium. They are also about 20 percent fat, with 3 percent saturated fat and the rest monounsaturated and polyunsaturated fat.

HISTORY

Soybeans made their first appearance in North America in 1765, when East India Company sailor Samuel Bowen brought them from China. He gave the seeds to Henry Yonge, a farmer in Georgia, who planted them and grew the first soybean crop on the continent. Bowen, Yonge, and others grew soy as animal feed, and Bowen made soy sauce from it that he exported for sale in England, but it took until the 1900s before Lafayette Mendel and Thomas Burr Osborne demonstrated that cooking soybeans turned them into a food palatable to humans.

In 1910, William Morse of the U.S. Department of Agriculture and his mentor, Charles V. Piper, introduced soybeans as a food crop to farmers in the Carolinas. Together they wrote *The Soybean*, a 1923 book filled with instructions for growing soy, recipes for cooking soybeans, and an extensive bibliography for farmers' reference. Morse's efforts to promote the soybean as a food product spanned his entire career, including his founding of the American Soybean Growers' Association. He spent considerable time in eastern Asia researching new varieties and growing practices and learning to produce the variety of foods the Chinese made from soy.

Meanwhile, the industry Morse had launched in North America by going door to door in North Carolina had grown beyond his expectations. Processing plants had sprung up in his two-year absence, and by 1929, U.S. farmers produced 9.4 million bushels of soybeans, a crop they had never planted just twenty years before. Exponential growth continued throughout the twentieth century, with 200 million bushels produced in 1949, rising into the billions by the end of the century, with soy crops blanketing more than seventy million acres of American farmland. Only a tiny fraction of this produce goes toward food, however—the bulk of the national soybean crop becomes the basis for many industrial products.

Tofu, also known as bean curd and now a staple of vegetarian and vegan diets, originated some two thousand years ago in China and spread throughout East Asian countries over the course of several centuries. It came to the fore in the United States in Japanese internment camps in the 1940s and slowly rose in popularity in Asian-American communities until it moved into the mainstream in the late twentieth century.

THE CONTROVERSY

On its face, soy seems to be a particularly healthful addition to a balanced diet. Research has shown that eating soy-based products as a hefty protein source can help lower blood sugar and contribute to a healthy heart. Soy contains many vitamins and minerals that the body needs for strength and proper functioning, and its fat content is well below meats and even some poultry. It provides fiber and essential amino acids and even antioxidants, which protect the body against cell damage.

So what could be wrong with soybeans? Soy contain isoflavones known as phytoestrogens, which can attach to estrogen receptors in the body and activate them. Some research suggests that these mimic estrogen, a hormone linked directly to fertility in women. One study of 315 women in an infertility program in Massachusetts indicated that women who reported that they regularly ate one or more of fifteen soy products specified by the researchers were 1.3–1.8 times more likely to conceive a child during infertility treatments than women who did not consume soy. However, earlier studies appear to indicate that eating 100 mg of isoflavones daily (eight or more servings of soy) can actually disrupt ovarian function and ovulation—though this is much more soy than most people would consume in a day in soy milk or in a meal of tofu or tempeh. A 2014 study (Jacobsen et al.) of 11,688 women between the ages of thirty and fifty for whom soy was a major part of their diet came to the same conclusion: Women who ate a lot of soy had more difficulty becoming pregnant than women who ate considerably less soy. With the understanding that many things can impact a woman's ability to conceive, the researchers concluded that "a high dietary isoflavone intake may have significant impact on fertility."

Most studies that examine women whose diets contain 10–25 mg of isoflavones a day, or one to four servings of soy foods, found that consuming this moderate amount of soy had no effect on ovulation or fertility. Soy's high content of phytoestrogens suggests, however, that eating more soy might benefit women beyond childbearing age who are experiencing the symptoms of menopause—especially hot flashes. Here again, conflicting research leaves us with no specific conclusion: Some studies suggest that taking extracted, synthesized soy isoflavone supplements can calm hot flashes and limit their frequency and even relieve other symptoms of menopause including depression, irritability, anxiety, joint pain, and vaginal dryness . . . and some research indicates that these supplements had no effect on these symptoms.

Perhaps the most hopeful benefit of eating more soy is the possibility that it helps reduce the risk of cancer. A number of studies have explored the links between soy consumption, isoflavones, and breast cancer survival. A meta-analysis (Qiu and Jiang, 2018) published in 2019 of twelve studies with a total of 37,275 subjects found that postmenopausal women who ate soy products regularly before their breast cancer diagnosis were more likely to survive breast cancer and less likely to have the cancer recur. Eating soy after diagnosis resulted in "no significant association" with breast cancer survival, and premenopausal women did not seem to derive the same benefit. A meta-analysis published in 2020 (Wei et al., 2020) involving 300,000 women in the China Kadoorie Biobank study suggests that both premenopausal and postmenopausal women may have gained more protection from cancer the more soy they ate, achieving up to a 27 percent lower risk of cancer. Randomized, double-blind studies are still required to determine if correlation does indeed mean causation in this case.

In addition, eating soy may be helpful to some people who have specific gut bacteria that turn soy into equol, a metabolite that may lower the levels of white matter lesions in the brains of elderly people. White matter lesions lead to cognitive decline and dementia, but people who can produce equol from soy have 50 percent fewer of these lesions, according to a study by Sekikawa et al., published in October 2020. The appropriate gut bacteria to accomplish this show up in about 70 percent of people in Japan, where the study took place; in America, however, fewer than a third of the population has these bacteria. The small study followed ninety-one elderly people for four years who were "cognitively normal" at the beginning of the study and then reconnected with them six to nine years later to take MRI and PET scans to see if they developed the white matter lesions. The people who produced more equol had fewer lesions in the follow-up. "We cannot prove that equol protects against dementia until we get a randomized clinical trial with sufficient evidence," Sekikawa cautioned.

FURTHER READINGS

George, Judy. "Soy Metabolite Tied to Dementia Risk Factors." *MedPage Today*, Oct. 22, 2020. Accessed Oct. 25, 2020. https://www.medpagetoday.com/neurology/dementia/89271

Jacobsen, Bjarne K., et al. "Soy Isoflavone Intake and the Likelihood of Every Becoming a Mother: The Adventist Health Study-2." *International Journal of Women's Health*, 2014, 6, 377–384. Accessed Oct. 20, 2020. https://www.ncbi.nlm.nih.gov/pmc/articles/PMC3982974/

Jefferson, Wendy. "Adult Ovarian Function Can Be Affected by High Levels of Soy." *Journal of Nutrition*, Dec. 2010, 140(12), 2322S–2325S. Accessed Oct. 20, 2020. https://www.ncbi.nlm.nih.gov/pmc/articles/PMC3139237/

Matias, Mariana; and Mark Ash. "Soybean Demand Projected to Grow in 2019/2020, But Record Inventories Dampen Prices." USDA Economic Research Service, Aug.

12, 2019. Accessed Oct. 20, 2020. https://www.ers.usda.gov/amber-waves/2019/august/soybean-demand-projected-to-grow-in-201920-but-record-inventories-dampen-prices/

Qiu, Shumin; and Jiang, Chongmin. "Soy and Isoflavones Consumption and Breast Cancer Survival and Recurrence: A Systematic Review and Meta-analysis." *European Journal of Nutrition*, Dec. 2019, 58(8), 3079–3090. Accessed Oct. 21, 2020. https://pubmed.ncbi.nlm.nih.gov/30382332/

Sekikawa, Akira, et al. "Associations of Equol-Producing Status with White Matter Lesion and Amyloid-ß Deposition in Cognitively Normal Elderly Japanese." *Translational Research and Clinical Intervention*, 2020, 6(1). Accessed Oct. 25, 2020. https://alz-journals.onlinelibrary.wiley.com/doi/full/10.1002/trc2.12089

Shurtleff, William; and Aoyagi, Akiko. "William J. Morse and Charles V. Piper: Work With Soy." SoyInfo Center, 2004. Accessed Oct. 20, 2020. https://www.soyinfocenter.com/HSS/morse_and_piper.php

Taku, Kyoto, et al. "Extracted or Synthesized Soybean Isoflavones Reduce Menopausal Hot Flash Frequency and Severity: Systematic Review and Meta-analysis of Randomized Control Trials." *Menopause*, July 2012, 19(7), 776–790. Accessed Oct. 20, 2020. https://pubmed.ncbi.nlm.nih.gov/22433977/

Vanegas, Jose C., et al. "Soy Food Intake and Treatment Outcomes of Women Undergoing Assisted Reproductive Technology." *Fertility and Sterility*, Mar. 2015, 103(3), 749–755. Accessed Oct. 20, 2020. https://www.ncbi.nlm.nih.gov/pmc/articles/PMC4346414/

Wei, Yuxia, et al. "Soy Intake and Breast Cancer Risk: A Prospective Study of 300,000 Chinese Women and a Dose-Response Meta-analysis." *European Journal of Epidemiology*, June 2020, 35(6), 567–578. Accessed Oct. 21, 2020. https://pubmed.ncbi.nlm.nih.gov/31754945/

Sugar Alcohols

WHAT ARE THEY?

Sugar alcohols (polyols), which are found in many fruits, berries, and vegetables and are extracted through a chemical process, are considered sugar substitutes. These are factory-produced for use in sweetening processed foods. Erythritol, hydrogenated starch hydrolysates (HSHs), isomalt, lactitol, maltitol, mannitol, sorbitol, and xylitol are all listed by the FDA as sugar alcohols. These are neither sugar nor alcohol—they are hybrids of both sugar and alcohol molecules, but they do not contain either and are safe for people who have issues with alcohol. They do add carbohydrates to food, so they can have an effect on caloric content and blood glucose.

CURRENT CONSUMPTION STATISTICS AND TRENDS

Globally, sugar alcohols were a $3.61 billion business in 2019. This market is expected to nearly double to $6.7 billion by 2027, but most of this growth comes from the use of sugar alcohols in hand sanitizers, not in food products. In fact, Fortune Business Insights reports that the use of sugar alcohols in foods dropped in the early 2020s, largely because of the reduction in sales of chewing gum, candies, and baked goods as people who lost income during the COVID-19 pandemic limited their grocery purchases to essentials.

NUTRITIONAL INFORMATION

Sugar alcohols in themselves provide no nutritional content. Their value comes from their use as a low-glycemic replacement for sugar, reducing the impact of some foods in contributing to obesity, metabolic syndrome, cardiovascular disease, and diabetes. Sugar alcohols provide about one-third to one-half fewer calories than sugar (about 2.6 calories per gram, while sugar is 4 calories per gram), but they convert to glucose more slowly than sugar does, so they require very little insulin to metabolize. This prevents spikes in blood sugar, making foods that contain sugar alcohols comparatively safe for diabetics.

As they are not readily available for home use, most consumers only encounter these sweeteners in processed foods like candies, baked goods, ice cream, and frozen confections, which may be high in calories and contain high levels of simple carbohydrates. In addition, sugar alcohols are difficult for the body to digest, so eating large amounts of products containing them can result in bloating, flatulence, and diarrhea.

HISTORY

Hermann Emil Fischer, a German scientist, made a landmark discovery in the development of carbohydrate chemistry in 1891, when he determined the formula that became known as the sugar family tree. In the course of his research, he obtained xylitol from berries by reducing D-xylose with sodium amalgamate. The magnitude of his discovery did not become apparent immediately, however—in fact, not until the 1970s did food manufacturers begin producing xylitol on a commercial scale, and then it became more in demand by the dental hygiene industry than food manufacturers, as xylitol turned out to be a natural cavity-fighting agent.

Fischer also discovered sorbitol in his experiments with glucose and sodium amalgamate, and in 1912, V. Ipatieff built on Fischer's research when he performed the first catalytic hydrogenation (addition of hydrogen atoms to a molecule) of sorbitol. Proof that this sweetener could be synthesized by industry led to interest from food manufacturers who improved on the process in 1925, and by the 1950s, sorbitol became an important ingredient in many foods. Further research found that it also serves as a stabilizer of humidity, increasing its value to the cosmetics industry and making it an ingredient in forming pharmaceutical tablets.

In the 1960s, HSHs had their origin at Lyckeby Starch, a Swedish company—in fact, the Lyckeby laboratory is credited with the development of most hydrogenated products. Maltitol also emerged there, synthesized using chromatography, a process of separating high-maltose glucose corn syrups into their individual components.

The youngest of the sugar alcohols, erythritol, occurs naturally in fruits—especially fermented fruits—and vegetables. It has no calories and does not produce the digestive issues that most sugar alcohols cause, making it particularly interesting to the food industry. It came into commercial use in the 1990s in Japan and has since become available worldwide, with Cargill as its prime manufacturer.

THE CONTROVERSY

Are sugar alcohols better than sugar? The answer to this depends on what consumers are willing to tolerate in exchange for enjoying the sweet taste of their favorite confection.

For the most part—with the exception of maltitol—sugar alcohols have a much lower glycemic index (GI) than sugar. The GI measures how quickly foods increase blood sugar levels, a critically important factor in controlling weight gain, metabolic syndrome, and diabetes. Several sugar alcohols have a GI of 0 or close to 0: erythritol, mannitol, and sucralose. Lactitol, sorbitol, and xylitol raise blood sugar slightly, while maltitol's GI is 36, which is still just over half the GI of sugar (65).

This makes some dieters think that foods that contain sugar alcohols can be consumed indiscriminately, in whatever amounts they choose. Most of the processed food products that contain sugar alcohols, however, are highly caloric in other ways. Sweets like cookies, cake, pie, and candies often contain other kinds of carbohydrates from wheat flour, corn syrup, and other ingredients, some of which can cause almost as much trouble to diabetics as sugar. These products may have fewer calories than those made with sugar, but they do not represent a free pass for bingeing. Consumers need to check labels for portion sizes and follow them carefully to enjoy the benefits of sugar alcohols' sweetness, lower calories, and lower GI.

Sugar alcohols (with the exception of erythritol) are fermentable oligo-, di-, monosaccharides, and polyols (FODMAPs), carbohydrates that resist digestion. This means that they do not get absorbed into the bloodstream, but continue to travel to the far reaches of the digestive system to feed the gut bacteria. Here they do the job of fueling the gut, which produces hydrogen gas. They also pull liquid from the rest of the body into the intestine, loosening bowel movements.

None of this is harmful, but it can be uncomfortable and embarrassing, and the resulting flatulence and diarrhea can make consumers think that sugar alcohols are making them sick. The symptoms are temporary and leave the body fairly rapidly. People with irritable bowel syndrome or other digestive diseases may want to avoid foods with sugar alcohols, however, as these symptoms can exacerbate an already uncomfortable situation.

FURTHER READINGS

Arrigoni, Eva, et al. "Human Gut Microbiota Does Not Ferment Erythritol." *British Journal of Nutrition*, Nov. 2005, 94(5), 643–646. Accessed Oct. 21, 2020. https://pubmed.ncbi.nlm.nih.gov/16277764/

"Eat Any Sugar Alcohol Lately?" Yale New Haven Health. Accessed Oct. 21, 2020. https://www.ynhh.org/services/nutrition/sugar-alcohol.aspx

Hyams, J.S. "Sorbitol Intolerance: An Unappreciated Cause of Functional Gastrointestinal Complaints." *Gastroenterology*, Jan. 1983, 84(1), 30–33. Accessed Oct. 21, 2020. https://pubmed.ncbi.nlm.nih.gov/6847853/

Leech, Joe. "Sugar Alcohols: Good or Bad?" Healthline, Sept. 19, 2018. Accessed Oct. 21, 2020. https://www.healthline.com/nutrition/sugar-alcohols-good-or-bad

Schiweck, Hubert, et al. "Sugar Alcohols." *Ullmann's Encyclopedia of Industrial Chemistry*, May 30, 2011. Accessed Oct. 21, 2020. https://onlinelibrary.wiley.com/doi/10.1002/14356007.a25_413.pub2

"Sugar Alcohols." U.S. Food and Drug Administration. Accessed Aug. 19, 2019. https://www.accessdata.fda.gov/scripts/InteractiveNutritionFactsLabel/sugar-alcohol.html

"Sugar Alcohol Market Size, Share & COVID-19 Impact Analysis By Type . . ." *Fortune Business Insights*, June 2020. Accessed Oct. 21, 2020. https://www.fortunebusinessinsights.com/sugar-alcohol-market-102956

Superfoods

WHAT ARE THEY?

Foods that are considered particularly nutritious and important to the human body may be categorized as superfoods by the media. No scientific criteria or government agencies qualify any food to rank above others as a superfood. Foods including acai berries, almonds, avocado, blueberries, broccoli, chia seeds, dark chocolate, garlic, green tea, kale, kefir, kombucha, mangosteen, olive oil, pomegranate, quinoa, salmon, seaweed, wheatgrass, and others have found their way into the superfood category, but some cycle off the list when exotic new foods emerge as potential superfood contenders. Some food manufacturers label their products as superfoods as a marketing tactic, whether or not they have the healthful qualities that others can claim.

CURRENT CONSUMPTION STATISTICS AND TRENDS

Despite the fairly flimsy categorization, superfoods represent big business. The global market for these foods reached $137 billion in 2018, and forecasters expect it to reach $204.6 billion by 2025. These statistics, computed by the market research firm Statista, measure the popularity of ancient grains, chia seeds, pulses (dry beans, seeds, lentils, and other legumes that grow in pods), seaweed, and kombucha. The focus on maintaining good health brought on by the COVID-19 pandemic encourages consumers to purchase healthier foods—good news for purveyors of these products.

NUTRITIONAL INFORMATION

The nutrients that may be available from superfoods vary according to the nature of the specific food, but most superfoods contain antioxidants, healthy fats, fiber, and a wide range of vitamins and minerals.

HISTORY

The earliest recorded use of the term "superfood" appears to be by the United Fruit Company during World War I, when the company imported a large number of bananas. To move this product quickly before it all spoiled, United Fruit published pamphlets describing the wealth of nutrients, the convenience, and the many uses bananas provided to the American household. When medical journals endorsed bananas as a superfood, including the claim that bananas might cure celiac disease (before the research that proved that gluten caused the illness), the label stuck, and bananas became the first food marketed for its supposed superpowers.

Many foods have received this title since then, but the arrival of the Internet and its ability to spread information worldwide in seconds allows word of each new food's magic to become big news at lightning speed. Blueberries, one of the lasting beneficiaries of the superfood label, rose to prominence in 1991 when the USDA and the National Institute on Aging published a ranking of foods with high levels of antioxidants, known at the time as fighters of free radicals, toxic molecules that can initiate disease. Blueberries topped the list, and claims began to circulate that these berries could fight anything from cancer to heart disease. The USDA later removed the database from its website because it did not take into account the many other functions antioxidants have in the body, but blueberries' reputation remained intact, and they persist as a darling of superfood followers decades after the initial ranking.

The value of the superfood label to food packagers has proven its worth many times over in the marketplace. In 2015, for example, Royal Hawaiian Macadamia Nut applied to the FDA for permission to say on its packaging that daily consumption of the nuts could reduce the risk of heart disease. The FDA reviewed the 81-page petition with its accounts of several studies, including one conducted by Hershey Corporation, makers of many chocolate candies including chocolate-covered macadamia nuts. The FDA finally gave permission in 2017 for the company to make a well-qualified claim, with this exact wording: "Supportive but not conclusive research shows that eating 1.5 ounces per day of macadamia nuts, as part of a diet low in saturated fat and cholesterol and not resulting in increased intake of saturated fat or calories, may reduce the risk of coronary heart disease."

It might seem on the surface that such a complex statement would barely catch the eyes of consumers, but Royal Hawaiian's publicity department did yeoman's work in getting the desired message out to the media. Sure enough, *Hawaii News Now* declared, "Go nuts, folks! FDA declares macadamia nuts heart healthy," and today many websites that provide nutritional information to consumers, from Healthline to the Mayo Clinic, have a page devoted to the benefits of eating macadamia nuts, including their impact in reducing cholesterol levels all on their own.

THE CONTROVERSY

With this long history of increased popularity of specific foods that may qualify for the superfood moniker, food companies continue to pay for research that gets their product on the list, and they back that research with publicity to be sure that consumers know all about the product's healthful benefits. Consumers who now sprinkle powdered goji berries over their yogurt, who suffer through bitter shots of wheatgrass juice at soft drink stands, and who add chia and flax seeds to their smoothies have experienced the power of this marketing, whether or not they gain the promised health benefits from consuming these foods.

"No single food can offer every single nutritional component or health benefit we need," said Northwestern Medicine dietitian Sarah Buytendorp in an article on the medical center's website. "Healthy eating is a pattern, and 'superfood' is a marketing term."

The term "superfood" has no official or scientific definition, making it very much subject to interpretation. Some of the foods that have earned the title truly have high concentrations of nutrients and other natural substances that contribute to human health—blueberries, for example, contain large concentrations of antioxidants, molecules that protect the body from cancer-causing free radicals. Pomegranates contain antioxidants as well, and an extensive study published in 2014 in *Advanced Biomedical Research* determined that its juice can indeed reduce oxidative stress and free radicals, and it can even help lower blood pressure and prevent the growth of carcinogenic cells.

Many foods have been elevated to superfood status because of one health claim or another, but the veracity of these claims still comes into question. For example, the website WildBlueberries.com, a marketing site for a blueberry grower and packager, states that a lab-testing procedure performed by a USDA researcher "found that a one-cup serving of Wild Blueberries has more total antioxidant capacity that twenty other fruits and veggies," with a list of some of the fruits these blueberries beat. Whether this is enough to fight cancer, however, is not specified . . . because the nine studies listed by the National Cancer Institute that have attempted to answer this question have been inconclusive. In fact, none of them found a lowered incidence of cancer from taking antioxidant supplements, which had even higher concentrations of antioxidants than those claimed by blueberry marketers.

In fact, most of the messages about superfoods come from the food producers, not from the scientific community. Some of these have research that backs up the substance of their claims, but they usually lack the information consumers need to add enough of the food to their diet to achieve the desired effect. The good news is that few, if any, of these foods are likely to have anything but a benefit if added to a person's dinner plate—but if consumers choose these foods because of their ability to ward off disease on their own, they are likely to be disappointed.

Much of this research can be deliberately misleading, noted acclaimed food science researcher Marion Nestle in an article in *The Atlantic* in 2018. "This kind of research is designed to produce results implying that people who eat this one food will be healthier and can forget about everything else in their diets," she said. "Research aimed at marketing raises questions about biases in design and interpretation, may create reputational risks for investigators, and reflects poorly on the integrity of nutrition science."

Medical professionals agree on one thing: No one food provides all of the nutrients people need to maintain good health. The U.S. dietary guidelines call for a largely plant-based diet full of fruits, vegetables, whole grains, beans, and nuts, with proteins from the low-fat dairy, lean meats, and fish categories; eating mostly unprocessed foods and skimping on salt and sugar serve as good ways to avoid cardiovascular disease, metabolic syndrome, diabetes, and other life-threatening illnesses that have their roots in a poor diet.

FURTHER READINGS

"Do Superfoods Exist?" *Northwestern Medicine*, 2020. Accessed Jan. 16, 2020. https://www.nm.org/healthbeat/healthy-tips/nutrition/superfoods-through-the-decades

"Go Nuts, Folks! FDA Declares Macadamia Nuts Heart Healthy." *Hawaii News Now*, July 24, 2017. Accessed Oct. 21, 2020. https://www.hawaiinewsnow.com/story/35960925/go-nuts-folks-fda-declares-macadamia-nuts-heart-healthy/

Nestle, Marion. "Superfoods Are A Marketing Ploy." *The Atlantic*, Oct. 23, 2018. Accessed Oct. 21, 2020. https://www.theatlantic.com/health/archive/2018/10/superfoods-marketing-ploy/573583/

"Superfoods or Superhype?" Harvard T.H. Chan School of Public Health. Accessed Oct. 21, 2020. https://www.hsph.harvard.edu/nutritionsource/superfoods/

Wanjek, Christopher. "What Are Superfoods?" *LiveScience*, Mar. 18, 2019. Accessed Oct. 21, 2020. https://www.livescience.com/34693-superfoods.html

Zarfeshany, Aida; Asgary, Sedigheh; and Javanmard, Shaghayegh Haghjoo. "Potent Health Effects of Pomegranate." *Advanced Biomedical Research*, 2014, 3(100). Accessed Jan. 16, 2020. https://www.ncbi.nlm.nih.gov/pmc/articles/PMC4007340/

Vegetable Oil

WHAT IS IT?

Vegetable oils are oils extracted from parts of a plant—a fruit, vegetable, grain, seed, or nut. They contain triglycerides, or fats, which makes them useful in cooking. By definition, oils are liquid at room temperature, which makes them different from butters and shortenings that are solid until heated.

Oils extracted from fruit include corn, olive, palm, and rice bran oil; those from seeds include canola, cottonseed, grapeseed, pumpkinseed, safflower, sesame, soybean, and sunflower oil. Almond, beech nut, Brazil nut, cashew, hazelnut, macadamia, pecan, pine nut, peanut, pistachio, and walnut oil are all extracted from ground nuts, which contain both saturated fat and monounsaturated and polyunsaturated fats.

CURRENT CONSUMPTION STATISTICS AND TRENDS

Palm, soybean, canola, and sunflower seed oil have the highest consumption worldwide, with uses both as food and for fuel and diesel production. Total global vegetable oil production in 2019–2020 reached 203.91 million metric tons, with palm oil representing 71.48 million metric tons of this total. Soybean oil comes in second at 55.46 million metric tons, and rapeseed (canola) oil ranks third, with 27.62 million tons.

NUTRITIONAL INFORMATION

On average, a tablespoon of vegetable oil provides 120 calories, all of which come from fat (14 g). Of this fat, 1–2 g is saturated fat; the rest is monounsaturated and polyunsaturated fat. Vegetable oils including soybean, corn, cottonseed, sunflower, peanut, sesame, and rice bran are also high in omega-6 fatty acids.

HISTORY

Vegetable oils became staples of the human diet thousands of years ago, when ancient cultures discovered that heating oily plants produced a liquid they could collect and use in cooking. Soy oil emerged in China and Japan by 2000 BC, while indigenous North Americans found that they could pound peanuts and sunflower seeds into a paste and boil it, skimming the oil that rose to the surface off the top for later use. Oils are mentioned repeatedly in the Old and New Testaments of the Judeo-Christian Bible, used as a sacrament in the early temples and for anointing and cleansing in the Gospels. On the African continent, people crushed coconut meat and palm kernels into a pulp, boiling this in water and collecting the resulting oil as it rose to the surface.

The need to increase production beyond personal use led to innovations in extracting the oil from plants. People in widely disparate countries came up with the same ideas independently, crushing large amounts of plant matter by grinding it between millstones or with an outsized mortar and pestle, placing the crushed material in shallow wicker baskets and stacking them on top of one another. The last step involved pressing out the oil using a lever or wedge press. In Greece and Rome, where many innovations took place, both societies developed the screw or winch to make the lever press easier to operate and more productive.

In the 1600s, inventors in Holland created the stamper press to extract more oil, a device that remained in use until the 1800s. English inventor John Smeaton came up with the roll mill in 1750, a more efficient way to press the plant material; another Englishman, Joseph Bramah, invented the hydraulic press and changed the way many industrial processes were achieved, including oil extraction. An American, V.D. Anderson, built a continuously operating cage press in 1876 that he called the Expeller, a name that stuck and became the trade name for his process. The Expeller directed the oil to drain out of slots in the sides of the press as a screw increased the pressure, allowing the process to continue even as operators collected the oil.

The use of solvents like benzene to extract the oil began in 1856 in England, a practice that has become the standard for obtaining as much oil as possible from the plant material. This method allows manufacturers to gather all but 0.5–2 percent of the oil in the material, a considerable improvement over early methods that only managed to obtain about 10 percent of the available oil from the crushed plants or seeds. The solvent (now hexane) is removed by distilling the oil, which brings all of the solvent to the top to evaporate. A stripping column gathers and removes whatever fraction of the solvent remains before the oil is refined for bottling.

THE CONTROVERSY

Replacing saturated fat in the human diet with polyunsaturated and monounsaturated fats has led to the popularity of vegetable oils over solid shortening, lard, and butter, saturated fats that increase cholesterol levels. Which oils are healthier and which oils we should avoid continue to be up for debate.

Some science points to omega-6 fatty acids, polyunsaturated fats found in nuts, seeds, and vegetable oils, as a healthful benefit to using these oils. Other studies suggest that an imbalance between omega-3 and omega-6 fatty acids can actually cause inflammation in the body, which can contribute to heart disease, diabetes, and other systemic issues.

The benefits of omega-3s have become well known among consumers, leading to increased consumption of fatty fish like salmon and mackerel, flaxseeds, walnuts, and other foods high in these fats. Omega-3s help the heart maintain its rhythm, calm inflammation, prevent blood clots inside blood vessels, and lower triglyceride levels. Omega-6s also provide benefits: They lower LDL cholesterol, raise HDL cholesterol, and improve the body's sensitivity to insulin, preventing blood sugar spikes and drops.

Some researchers argue that omega-6 fats also can have negative effects. The human body has the ability to convert omega-6 fats into arachidonic acid, which molecules need to create inflammation and blood clots. Other studies note that the body can use arachidonic acid to do exactly the opposite, reducing inflammation and helping blood move smoothly through arteries and veins.

To examine the issue as closely as possible, the American Heart Association brought together nine scientists from universities throughout the United States in 2007 to review all of the research to date on omega-6 fatty acids. The journal *Circulation* published their findings in 2009: They determined that eating more omega-6 fats reduced inflammation markers or had no effect on them, and heart disease rates dropped in populations that consumed more omega-6 fats. In fact, one meta-analysis showed that replacing saturated fat with omega-6 fats actually reduced the risk of heart attacks by 24 percent.

Additional studies, including a meta-analysis of eleven studies published in the *American Journal of Clinical Nutrition*, showed positive results in replacing saturated fats with polyunsaturated fats, especially when compared to replacing saturated fats with monounsaturated fats or carbohydrates. The American Heart Association embraced the use of polyunsaturated fats with omega-3 and omega-6 fatty acids as the gold standard for heart health. The organization recommends maintaining a balance of the two omegas for the best health outcomes.

This may sound like settled science, but authorities still disagree on whether omega-6 fats are more beneficial or more harmful to the body. A study published in *Prostaglandins, Leukotrienes and Essential Fatty Acids* in May 2018 called the relationship between omega-3 and omega-6 fats and inflammation "complex and still not properly understood." The study makes reference to research that shows a correlation between omega-6 levels and inflammation and other studies that demonstrate that omega-6 fats actually reduce inflammation. A 2016 study (Simopoulos) suggests that eating more foods high in omega-6 fats and less food with omega-3 fats upsets the balance between the two fats, which then triggers obesity. "It is quite probable that gene [polyunsaturated fatty acid] interactions induced by the modern Western diet are differentially driving the risk of diseases of inflammation (obesity, diabetes, atherosclerosis and cancer) in diverse populations," the report said.

A September 2020 study published in *Nutrients* came to the conclusion that the 1:1 ratio of omega-3 fats to omega-6 fats in a healthy diet can have a positive effect in fighting inflammation, preventing diseases including obesity and colorectal cancer, among others. "Appropriate dietary intervention has primarily relevance in the prevention and treatment of obesity in that it maintains the efficiency of key signaling pathways and avoids long term/chronic inflammatory states," the paper concluded.

While the controversy continues, science appears to draw consensus about one issue: The balance between these two fatty acids plays an important role in gaining the greatest benefit from consuming them. As the human body cannot make its own omega-3 or omega-6 fats and must acquire them from food, choosing a diet that includes sources of both fats may have positive effects. Vegetable oils as a whole provide omega-6 fats, so omega-3s need to come from other foods.

FURTHER READINGS

Caporuscio, Jessica. "What Are the Most Healthful Oils?" *Medical News Today*, Mar. 30, 2019. Accessed Oct. 22, 2020. https://www.medicalnewstoday.com/articles/324844

"Cooking Oil." *Encyclopedia.com*, Oct. 3, 2020. Accessed Oct. 22, 2020. https://www.encyclopedia.com/manufacturing/news-wires-white-papers-and-books/cooking-oil

D'Angelo, Stefania, et al. "Omega-3 and Omega-6 Polyunsaturated Fatty Acids, Obesity and Cancer." *Nutrients*, Sept. 2020, 12(9), 2751. Accessed Oct. 22, 2020. https://www.ncbi.nlm.nih.gov/pmc/articles/PMC7551151/

Hooper, Lee, et al. "Reduction in Saturated Fat Intake for Cardiovascular Disease." *Cochrane Database System Review*, May 19, 2020, 5(5), CDO11737. Accessed Oct. 22, 2020. https://pubmed.ncbi.nlm.nih.gov/26068959/

Innes, Jacqueline K.; and Calder, Philip C. "Omega-6 Fatty Acids and Inflammation." *Prostaglandins, Leukotrienes and Essential Fatty Acids*, May 2018, 132, 41–48. Accessed Oct. 22, 2020. https://www.sciencedirect.com/science/article/abs/pii/S0952327818300747

"No Need to Avoid Health Omega-6 Fats." Harvard Health Publishing, Harvard Medical School, Aug. 20, 2019. Accessed Oct. 22, 2020. https://www.health.harvard.edu/newsletter_article/no-need-to-avoid-healthy-omega-6-fats

Shahbandeh, M. "Consumption of Vegetable Oils Worldwide From 2013/14 to 2019/2020." Statista, May 19, 2020. Accessed Oct. 22, 2020. https://www.statista.com/statistics/263937/vegetable-oils-global-consumption/

Simopoulos, Artemis P. "An Increase in the Omega-6/Omega-3 Fatty Acid Ration Increases the Risk for Obesity." *Nutrients*, Mar. 2016, 8(3), 128. Accessed Oct. 22, 2020. https://www.ncbi.nlm.nih.gov/pmc/articles/PMC4808858/

Wine

WHAT IS IT?

An alcoholic beverage made from fermenting grape juice, wine is the result of adding yeast to the juice to convert it to ethanol, carbon dioxide, and heat. Different grapes create different kinds of wines: white, red, rosé, sparkling, and sweet or dessert wine.

CURRENT CONSUMPTION STATISTICS AND TRENDS

According to the Wine Institute, U.S. residents consume an average of 2.95 gallons of wine annually (with the understanding that many people do not drink wine). This resulted in sales of 966 million gallons of wine in 2018. Sales of wine produced in California alone topped 275.6 million cases in 2019, with an estimated retail value of $43.6 billion. Washington State, the nation's second largest wine region, produces 17.7 million cases annually for $8.4 billion, and New York wines add $6.65 billion, with production of twenty-eight million gallons at 470 wineries in 2019.

NUTRITIONAL INFORMATION

A 5-ounce glass of wine contains about 120 calories, almost all of which comes from alcohol, and 1–4 g of carbohydrates. Red wine contains 1–2 g of carbohydrates extracted from the skin and seeds of the grapes; while white wine may contain no carbohydrates at all. Dry sparkling wines may contain no carbohydrates, while sweeter sparkling wines can have as much as 6 g of carbs per glass. Sweet wines like port and sauterne retain more sugar and are therefore higher in calories and carbs, though a serving may be as small as 2 ounces. The smaller glass size keeps the calories down to about 100 and limits the carbs to 4 g or less.

Wines also provide small amounts of minerals including manganese, potassium, iron, phosphorus, and B vitamins.

HISTORY

In 2007, researchers at the University of California at Los Angeles (UCLA), conducting an archaeological dig in Armenia, discovered what turned out to be the oldest winery in the world. Dating back to 4100 BC, the winery in a cave contained grape seeds and petrified vines, the remains of grapes in a primitive wine press, a fermentation vat made of clay, and bits of pottery soaked with wine.

Before this find, archaeologists believed that wine originated in ancient Egypt around 3100 BC, based on the Egyptians' use of a wine-like beverage made from red grapes, which they employed in ceremonial rites because it looked like blood. Visiting Phoenicians learned of the wine and took the knowledge with them, becoming the first civilization to cultivate grapes for winemaking. They brought it with them in their travels throughout the region, expanding interest in the fermented beverage among other cultures.

The discovery of a wine cellar in Israel marked another milestone in wine production: The storage facility, dating to about 1700 BC, held vessels that could have stored as much as 500 gallons of wine—enough to fill 3,000 of today's bottles. A few hundred years later, the Phoenicians crossed the Mediterranean Sea and began trading with people in Greece and Italy, widening the territory in which wine could be cultivated. They also brought wine to the Jewish people of the Middle East, who began using it in religious ceremonies.

As Greece's empire grew, each new colony received its own grapevines for planting, and the Greeks even named a god of wine, Dionysus, within their pantheon. Soon they realized that the southern tip of Italy provided fine grape-growing soil and weather conditions. To this day, some of the world's finest wines come from this region, as well as from farther north in Italy, where the Romans made wine a central part of their culture and named their own god, Bacchus, as its patron.

The rise of the Roman Empire brought the pleasures of wine to people across Europe, establishing some of the most productive vineyards in the world in France, Spain, Germany, and Portugal. By AD 380, when the Romans adopted Christianity as their official religion and became the heart of the Catholic Church, wine had become part of the sacraments, and the church itself turned to wine cultivation and production as a central mission.

When Christopher Columbus accidentally sailed into the New World in 1492, his expedition brought wine with them; soon the conquistadors followed, and their travels across South America broadened the distribution of wines into an unexplored region. Missionaries planted vineyards to supply the wine for Communion, beginning what would become an important winegrowing region in Chile and Argentina. Not until 1619 would winemaking reach North America, when the French began cultivating grapes in Virginia, but the Puritans to the north and south turned up their noses at alcoholic beverages, so the enterprise fizzled. When Thomas Jefferson became the first U.S. minister to France in 1785, he found himself smitten by French Bordeaux and Burgundy wines and brought grapevines back to Virginia with him, determined to found a new industry there.

On the west coast, Father Junipero Serra arrived from Spain in 1769 to found his mission in San Diego, bringing grapevines to plant what became California's first vineyard. Franciscan monks found their way to the Napa Valley in 1805 and established Sonoma's first winery. Prospectors from the eastern United States came to California to seek their fortune in 1849, bringing their favorite wines with them, including a variety from Croatia called Zinfandel that turned out to be well suited to the Napa climate. It has since become one of California's most celebrated grapes.

Today wines are big business in the United States, with three major wine regions in California, Washington, and New York producing the most cases and varieties. Virginia continues to produce wines as well, and every state in the country has its own vintners, some of whom experiment with fruits other than grapes and produce all sorts of interesting beverages.

THE CONTROVERSY

Is wine good for you or not? The question arose in the late 1980s when scientists studying longevity in various cultures came upon the French, whose diet contains a great deal of butter, cheese, and other saturated fats, but who have a particularly low instance of heart disease (CHD). Serge Renaud, a scientist from Bordeaux, France, coined the phrase "French Paradox" for this. Renaud and his team concluded that what became known as the Mediterranean diet—high not only in fats but also in omega-3 fatty acids and other antioxidants—produced the remarkable effect of lowering overall LDL cholesterol and protecting the heart. An important component of this diet, they added, was "moderate consumption" of red wine.

This study piqued the interest of the CBS news program *60 Minutes*, which aired a segment about it that emphasized red wine's key role. The program's impact on the American dieters' psyche cannot be overstated: People rushed to stores to buy red wine and began to incorporate it into their daily lives.

What could be the magic element in red wine that caused this remarkable health in France? Scientists began to search for the answer, and they soon centered their investigation on resveratrol, an antimicrobial antioxidant found in the skin of grapes, where it protects the flesh of the fruit from parasites. Jang et al. (1997) reported on their work in extracting and purifying this substance and testing it in a laboratory—but on cancer rather than CHD, giving it to mice with breast cancer at three stages of development. The result: Resveratrol slowed the growth of the cancer cells. "These data suggest that resveratrol, a common constituent of the human diet, merits investigation as a potential cancer chemopreventive agent in humans," their paper concluded.

Their work, published in *Science*, caused another sensation in the popular press, triggering a further boom in the wine industry and leading many people to turn to the fermented grape in hopes that it would protect them from cancer and other potential threats to their health. One study does not usually establish a scientific fact on its own, but subsequent studies did produce similar results, including a 2001 paper (Waffo-Téguo et al.) that tested several substances in red wine for their ability to reduce cancer risk. They found that a second substance, *trans*-astringin, also prohibited the formation of lesions in mice with breast cancer. At the same time, some studies found that resveratrol had no effect on cancer growth, leaving the door open to additional research to determine if the substance affects some cancers, but not others.

What about heart disease? Studies suggest that if wine has any positive effect on the heart, it comes from the alcohol itself. In fact, ten studies have examined the effects of moderate consumption of alcohol on the heart, and three found that wine does indeed improve heart health . . . but three more studies said beer had a stronger effect, and three more suggested that liquor had more effect that wine. All of these emphasized that drinking in moderation—one glass of wine, one beer, or one beverage of distilled spirits—might produce the desired effect. Drinking in excess, however, did not provide positive results and in fact has a number of negative consequences.

Scientists investigating the role of red wine continue to disagree on whether it can indeed lower cholesterol and improve heart health. While we cannot be sure that resveratrol is the true answer to the French Paradox, there is certainly no harm in enjoying a glass of red wine with dinner, knowing that there may be a legitimate health benefit in doing so.

FURTHER READINGS

Cazentre, Don. "How Big Is New York's Wine Business? Inside the Numbers." *NewYork-Upstate.com*, Jan. 29, 2020. Accessed Oct. 22, 2020. https://www.newyorkupstate.com/wine-tours/2020/01/how-big-is-new-yorks-wine-business-inside-the-numbers.html

Das, D.K., et al. "Cardioprotection of Red Wine: Role of Polyphenolic Antioxidants." *Drugs Under Experimental and Clinical Research*, 1999, 25(2–3), 115–120. Accessed Oct. 22, 2020. https://pubmed.ncbi.nlm.nih.gov/10370873/

"How Wine Colonized the World." *VinePair*. Accessed Oct. 22, 2020. https://vinepair.com/wine-colonized-world-wine-history/#0

Jang, M., et al. "Cancer Chemopreventive Activity of Resveratrol, a Natural Product Derived From Grapes." *Science*, Jan. 10, 1997, 275(5297), 218–220. Accessed Oct. 22, 2020. https://pubmed.ncbi.nlm.nih.gov/8985016/

"Stats and Facts." *Washington State Wine*. Accessed Oct. 22, 2020. https://www.washingtonwine.org/wine/facts-and-stats/state-facts

Waffo-Téguo, P., et al. "Potential Cancer-Chemopreventive Activities of Wine Stilbenoids and Flavans Extracted From Grape (*Vitis vinifera*) Cell Cultures." *Nutrition and Cancer*, 2001, 40(2), 173–179. Accessed Oct. 22, 2020. https://pubmed.ncbi.nlm.nih.gov/11962253/

"Wine 4,100 BC—World's Oldest Winery Discovered." Science 2.0, Jan. 11, 2011. Accessed Oct. 22, 2020. https://www.science20.com/news_articles/wine_4100_bc_worlds_oldest_winery_discovered

"Wine Nutrition Facts." *Wine.com*. Accessed Oct. 22, 2020. https://www.wine.com/content/landing/nutrition#

"Wine Statistics." The Wine Institute. Accessed Oct. 22, 2020. https://wineinstitute.org/our-industry/statistics/

Xanthan Gum

WHAT IS IT?

Derived from sugar fermented by the bacterium *Xanthomonas campestris*, the soluble fiber known as xanthan gum serves as a thickening agent when added to liquid. Gluten-free bakers use it to replace the gluten that normally binds baked goods together. Salad dressings, fruit juices, packaged soups, ice cream, sauces, gravy, syrups, and some low-fat foods may also list xanthan gum among their ingredients. Many nonfood products including paint, grout, oven and toilet bowl cleaners, adhesives, fungicides and herbicides, toothpaste, lotions, shampoo, and others rely on xanthan gum as a binding agent and thickener.

CURRENT CONSUMPTION STATISTICS AND TRENDS

The global xanthan gum market reached $960 million in 2019 and continues to grow at a rate of 6 percent annually. The increase in people diagnosed with one of the gluten intolerance illnesses, coupled with popular demand for gluten-free products, fueled the growth of xanthan gum's market in the 2010s; this is expected to continue for the foreseeable future. The food and beverage market represents about 40 percent of xanthan gum's total sales, with the oil and gas, cosmetics, pharmaceuticals, and other industrial markets buying the rest.

NUTRITIONAL INFORMATION

Xanthan gum does not provide any nutrients to the human body. As a soluble fiber, it cannot break down in the digestive process and is expelled as waste.

HISTORY

Allene Rosalind Jeanes, a chemical researcher in the USDA Northern Regional Research Lab in Peoria, Illinois, discovered xanthan gum in the early 1960s in her work with natural polysaccharides (sugars). The resulting substance came to the attention of CP Kelco, a subsidiary of J.M. Huber Corporation, which brought it into commercial production under the trade name Kelzan. In 1968, the FDA approved it for use in food, classifying it as GRAS. It soon became a widespread food additive and made its way into many other industries because of its ease of use and dependable ability to serve as a binder and thickener.

THE CONTROVERSY

Today consumers can buy xanthan gum in the gluten-free section of many supermarkets and specialty grocery stores to use in baking. Some users become concerned, however, when eating bread or muffins they made with it leads to digestive cramps, flatulence, an increase in bowel movements, and diarrhea.

These symptoms do not mean that xanthan gum makes people sick. Xanthan gum is a soluble fiber, meaning that it cannot be digested by the human digestive system. It mixes with water and forms a gel, which moves out of the system of its own accord. Most people do not experience anything unpleasant unless they consume a large amount of xanthan gum—more than 15 g or much more than a sandwich made with gluten-free bread or a single muffin contains. Studies to determine any harmful effects called xanthan gum "a highly effective laxative agent," but found nothing more sinister than that. Some people may be more sensitive to this soluble fiber than others, as xanthan gum is made from sugar that may come from wheat, corn, dairy (lactose), or soy. People with a wheat allergy, lactose intolerance, or a soy allergy may need to avoid products that contain this gum, as the digestive issues it creates may be much more severe.

For most people, consuming xanthan gum produces no effect at all—no added calories, no digestive discomfort—making it a neutral experience. Some small studies in the 1980s, however, endeavored to determine if this ingredient may actually have a positive effect on health. In one such study (Osilesi et al., 1985), nine diabetic and four nondiabetic people ate a muffin provided by the researchers every day for twelve weeks. In the first 6 weeks, they received muffins with no xanthan gum in them, and in the second 6 weeks, the muffins contained 12 g of xanthan gum (which is a lot of xanthan gum). The researchers took blood samples at the beginning and end of the study and found that during the 6 weeks of eating muffins with a significant amount of xanthan gum, the subjects had lowered glucose levels. This may have been connected, at least in part, to the feeling of fullness the xanthan gum-laden muffins caused in the patients' digestive systems, which led to fewer snacks throughout the rest of the day.

Subsequent studies of xanthan gum as effective against high blood glucose did not emerge until many years later. In 2016, Fuwa et al. conducted a study in which they tested different combinations of xanthan gum and rice to see how they would affect blood sugar levels. The researchers found that adding xanthan gum while the rice cooked suppressed blood glucose levels fifteen and thirty minutes after the subjects ate the rice, and that their blood sugar was significantly lower in the group that consumed xanthan gum in their rice than in the group that just ate rice. They also determined that eating xanthan gum added to food was more effective than just taking xanthan gum (presumably in tablet form) before or after the rice meal.

In 2018, Tanaka et al. conducted a controlled clinical trial of xanthan gum on human subjects after another study showed that consuming it lowered blood glucose in rats. In the 2018 trial, the subjects fasted for twelve hours and then took a nutrient that contained xanthan gum at 9 a.m., while the control group took the same nutrient that did not contain the gum. The researchers then measured the subjects' blood glucose at regular intervals and found that the group that had taken xanthan gum had significantly lower blood sugar than the control group. They concluded that xanthan gum inhibits blood glucose in humans.

The research looks promising, but there just is not very much of it. Many studies have involved xanthan gum over the last decade, but the vast majority of these deal with industrial uses for this soluble fiber, not with its effects on the human body. For now, food manufacturers and other sponsors of research appear to be content with the knowledge that xanthan gum can be used safely as a food additive, with its additional benefits to be taken advantage of at some unspecified later date.

FURTHER READINGS

Daly, J.; Tomlin, J.; and Read, N.W. "The Effect of Feeding Xanthan Gum on Colonic Function in Man: Correlation with In Vitro Determinants of Bacterial Breakdown." *British Journal of Nutrition*, May 1993, 69(3), 897–902. Accessed Oct. 25, 2020. https://pubmed.ncbi.nlm.nih.gov/8329363/

Fuwa, Masako, et al. "Effect of Xanthan Gum on Blood Sugar Level After Cooked Rice Consumption." *Food Science and Technology Research*, Feb. 2016, 22(1), 117–126.

Accessed Oct. 25, 2020. https://www.researchgate.net/publication/296472055_Effect_of_Xanthan_Gum_on_Blood_Sugar_Level_after_Cooked_Rice_Consumption
Osilesi, O., et al. "Use of Xanthan Gum in Dietary Management of Diabetes Mellitus." *American Journal of Clinical Nutrition*, Oct. 1985, 42(4), 597–603. Accessed Oct. 25, 2020. https://pubmed.ncbi.nlm.nih.gov/4050722/
Tanaka, Hiroshi, et al. "The Addition of Xanthan Gum to Enteral Nutrition Suppresses Postprandial Glycemia in Humans." *Journal of Nutritional Science and Vitaminology*, 2018, 64(4), 284–286. Accessed Oct. 25, 2020. https://pubmed.ncbi.nlm.nih.gov/30175792/

Glossary

α-linolenic acid (ALA) A beneficial omega-3 fatty acid that may lower the risk of cardiovascular disease and slow down cancer cells' growth rate.

Alkaloid Compounds in plants that contain nitrogen, that do not break down in water, but do break down in alcohol, and that produce some effect on the human body. Nicotine, morphine, and quinine are all alkaloids.

Amino acids The basic molecules that form proteins and contain hydrogen, carbon, oxygen, and nitrogen.

Angiogenesis The formation of new blood vessels required for new fat tissue or cancerous tumors to grow.

Anthocyanins Antioxidants that lower cholesterol levels and encourage blood sugar to metabolize.

Antibiotics Chemical substances produced by microorganisms or fungi that can inhibit the growth of bacteria or that can destroy bacteria.

Antioxidant Organic substances or enzymes that can counteract the effects of oxidation in people or animals.

Arachidonic acid An essential fatty acid required for muscle movement, blood flow, and other functions.

Atherosclerosis A disease that results from the formation of plaque deposits inside arteries.

Bacteria One-celled organisms involved in infectious disease, fermentation, putrefaction (rot), and other positive and negative processes within and outside of the body.

Brachial artery The major blood vessel in the upper arm.

Carbohydrate The starch, sugar, and fiber found in many foods, including grains, fruits, and vegetables.

Carcinogen Substances that contribute to the growth of cancerous cells.

Catechin An antioxidant substance that helps protect cells from damage caused by free radicals.

Cholesterol A substance made by the liver and required by the body to protect cell membranes, detoxify the bloodstream, synthesize sex hormones, and produce bile in the liver. Too much cholesterol can produce hardening of the arteries, preventing blood flow and leading to blood clots, heart attack, and stroke.

Cohort study This study follows a specific group to determine its risk factors for a disease, condition, or other result. The study introduces a variable, which becomes a risk factor with a potential outcome. The researchers then monitor the cohort's compliance with the study variable, collect data, and determine the effect of the variable.

Conjugated linoleic acid (CLA) A nutrient that can lower the risk of type 2 diabetes, heart disease, and cancer in the human body.

Double blind A research study in which neither the subjects nor the scientists know which subjects have received the medication or substance being tested and which have not. This prevents subjective or even unconscious bias in the course of the study.

Electrolytes Substances that produce electrical impulses between nerves to enable nerves and muscles to function.

Endothelial cells Cells that line all blood vessels throughout the body.

Enzyme Proteins from living cells that can make chemical changes happen, such as digestion.

Ester A chemical compound derived from an acid; many of these create the fragrances of essential oils.

Fatty acids Acids with long hydrocarbon chains that bond to glycerol to form a fat.

Flavonoids Antioxidants found in tea, red wine, fruits, and vegetables. Flavonoids are made up of two aromatic rings linked by a carbon bridge.

FODMAP Fermentable oligo-, di-, monosaccharides, and polyols, carbohydrates that resist digestion and provide fuel to gut bacteria without raising calorie levels.

Glucose A sugar that occurs in the human body and serves as its chief source of energy.

Glucosinolates Compounds that give vegetables a bitter taste when chewed.

GRAS Generally Regarded As Safe, as determined by the U.S. Food and Drug Administration to classify ingredients for use in processed foods. It signifies that when used in the ways intended, there are no known harmful effects of adding the ingredient to foods.

Hydrocarbons Compounds that contain only hydrogen and carbon, including methane, acetylene, and benzene.

Hydrogenated Combined with hydrogen to create a saturated compound and increase its melting point.

Hydrolyzed Mixed with water.

Hypertension High blood pressure.

Inflammation A process in which white blood cells protect the body from bacteria, viruses, and other invaders. In some diseases, inflammation takes place when there are no invaders, creating a chronic condition that can be harmful to the body.

Isoflavones Estrogen produced by legume plants that may lower cholesterol, fight cancer, and ease symptoms of menopause.

Isothiocyanates Compounds that keep cancer cells from dividing.

Lipids Fats that work with proteins and carbohydrates to form the structure of living cells.

Literature review A report usually conducted by a panel of researchers who review all of the studies on a specific topic and compile a report for publication.

Macronutrients The three ways that the body gains its primary resources of nutrition and energy starch, protein, and fat.

Meta-analysis A report or study that combines data from a number of already completed studies to arrive at a conclusion.

Metabolic syndrome An increase in blood glucose, cholesterol, blood pressure, and other issues that can eventually lead to heart attack, stroke, and diabetes.

Metabolite A substance that results from a metabolic process, for example, producing energy for the body to function.

Methylxanthines A class of drugs produced naturally and used to treat asthma, emphysema, chronic bronchitis, and other airway issues.

Microbiome The bacteria and other microorganisms in the gut, which are necessary for digestion and other bodily functions.

Monounsaturated fat One of the dietary fats required by the human body for proper functioning; unsaturated fats are liquid at room temperature.

Oleic acid An omega-9 fatty acid found in olive oil that promotes the reproduction of a cell molecule that keeps cancer proteins from developing and interferes with pathways between cells that allow cancer cells to reproduce. It also helps reduce the decline of cognitive function in older adults.

Omega-3 fatty acids Healthy polyunsaturated fats that do not occur naturally in the human body, but are known to reduce heart disease risk factors, fight inflammation, improve mental health, fight age-related dementia and Alzheimer's disease, and even help prevent cancer. They must be obtained by consuming foods that contain them.

Organic Grown and processed according to guidelines set by the U.S. Department of Agriculture for use of natural substances and farming methods.

Organochlorines A large group of synthetic pesticides that contain aromatic, chlorinated molecules.

Peer-reviewed The process of having several scientists in the same field review a study to determine the credibility of the results based on the methods used to conduct it, any relevant conflicts of interest, or other factors that may have distorted or affirmed the results. Peer review gives credibility to studies published in scientific journals.

pH Literally "power of hydrogen," pH is a scale that specifies the acidity or basicity of a liquid. Acidic liquids have a lower pH than basic liquids.

Phenolic compounds Antioxidants that may help guard against cancer and other diseases.

Phytochemicals Compounds that protect the body from diseases.

Phytoestrogens Isoflavones that can attach to estrogen receptors in the body and activate them. Some research suggests that these mimic estrogen, a hormone linked directly to fertility in women.

Phytosterols A compound that comes from plants, which can be used to lower blood cholesterol levels by competing with dietary cholesterol for absorption in the bloodstream.

Polyphenols Antioxidants that help reduce inflammation throughout the body and protect cells from damage, making them protectors against the spread of cancer.

Polysaccharide A carbohydrate that consists of multiple sugar molecules that have bonded together.

Polyunsaturated fat The "good" kind of dietary fat, found in both plants and animals and required by the body for proper functioning.

Randomized trial This kind of study assigns subjects randomly to either an experimental group or a control group. The experimental group tests whatever the variable is—a new drug, a specific diet, a practice like exercise or therapy—while the control group does something else or does nothing at all. This allows the researchers to determine if the specific variable has an effect on the experimental group, in comparison to those who did not have that variable.

Saturated fat Fat that contains fatty acid molecules that are not double-bonded. Saturated fats are solid at room temperature and must be heated to become liquid, and they raise blood cholesterol.

Soluble fiber Fiber that attracts water in the digestive system and turns to gel, slowing digestion.

Trans fats Fats created by an industrial process so that they retain their solid consistency at room temperature. These fats raise the body's bad (LDL) cholesterol while suppressing the good (HDL) cholesterol.

Triglycerides Fats formed from glycerol and three groups of fatty acids; high levels of triglycerides in the blood increase the risk of stroke.

Urinalysis Medical tests that involve analyzing urine for the presence of specific bacteria, blood, and other compounds that may indicate illness or disease.

Directory of Resources

American Cancer Society Guidelines for Diet and Physical Activity: https://www.cancer.org/healthy/eat-healthy-get-active/acs-guidelines-nutrition-physical-activity-cancer-prevention/guidelines.html

American Diabetes Association Nutrition site: https://www.diabetes.org/nutrition

American Heart Association Healthy Eating: https://www.heart.org/en/healthy-living/healthy-eating

Choose MyPlate: USDA healthy eating guide: https://www.fns.usda.gov/program/choose-myplate

Food Politics, website of author, professor, policy advisor, and food industry influence researcher Marion Nestle: https://www.foodpolitics.com

National Institute on Aging Healthy Eating resources: https://www.nia.nih.gov/health/healthy-eating

Nutrition and Healthy Eating, Mayo Clinic: https://www.mayoclinic.org/healthy-lifestyle/nutrition-and-healthy-eating/basics/nutrition-basics/hlv-20049477

The Nutrition Source, Harvard T.H. Chan School of Public Health: https://www.hsph.harvard.edu/nutritionsource/

Nutrition Strategies and Resources, a portal to government initiatives and information sources: https://www.cdc.gov/nccdphp/dnpao/state-local-programs/nutrition.html

President's Council on Sports, Fitness & Nutrition: https://www.hhs.gov/fitness/index.html

Substances Added to Food database, U.S. Food and Drug Administration: https://www.accessdata.fda.gov/scripts/fdcc/?set=FoodSubstances

U.S. Centers for Disease Control and Prevention Newsroom, for information on current outbreaks, food safety releases, and other news: https://www.cdc.gov/media/archives.html?Sort=Article%20Date%3A%3Adesc

U.S. Department of Agriculture Food Safety and Nutrition: https://www.usda.gov/topics/food-and-nutrition

U.S. Food and Drug Administration: Generally Regarded as Safe (GRAS): https://www.fda.gov/food/food-ingredients-packaging/generally-recognized-safe-gras

USDA FoodData Central: https://fdc.nal.usda.gov

USDA Nutrition.gov, offering "credible information to help you make healthful eating choices": https://www.nutrition.gov

Index

About the Author

RANDI MINETOR, MA, is a medical journalist and the author of *Medical Tests in Context: Innovations and Insights* and *Blowing Up: The Psychology of Conflict*, as well as more than 60 books on nature, travel, and general interest topics. She writes for *Western New York Physician* magazine, and she has served as a principal writer of patient, consumer, and doctor-to-doctor materials for the University of Rochester Medical Center. She is a graduate of the University of Rochester and the University at Buffalo. Follow her on Facebook @minetorbooks, on Twitter @rminetor, and on Instagram @writerrandi.